"The timing and content in this book could not be better! As we apply lessons learned from the pandemic, public health practitioners need to be able to blend their public health expertise with knowledge of complex and often competing systems. This book provides the tools that are needed, all in one place, to support leading healthy systems level change. I recommend it to students, faculty, and public health practitioners who need a fresh, new approach to their leadership development."

Kaye Bender, PhD, RN, FAAN
Executive Director
Mississippi Public Health Association

"I am excited and grateful for this book, a huge step towards building capacity for systems change in public health and beyond. The book thoughtfully combines well respected and diverse bodies of work, making them accessible and applicable to different levels of systemic intervention. Each chapter balances solid framing with a generous amount of detailed and applied cases and tools. This is the type of integration that the field of systems change has been looking for!"

Marta Ceroni
Co-Director
Academy for Systems Change

"Given the strong correlation between income and wealth as a predictor of better health outcomes and more than 100 million people in America experiencing economic insecurity, this book is critical to overcoming the harmful design challenges embedded within our laws, regulations, customs, and institutions. This book equips leaders to see systems in their entirety and transform them. It also provides a path forward for marshaling the courage to create a just and fair society—one where all people can participate, prosper, and reach their full potential."

Michael McAfee, EdD
President and CEO
PolicyLink

"This is an essential book for all leaders in public health. If public health as an industry is really invested in health and racial equity, it's imperative that we embrace systems change thinking and interventions. This is the roadmap we need, for how to do just that."

Lauren R. Powell, PhD, MPA
President and CEO
The Equitist

LEADING SYSTEMS CHANGE IN PUBLIC HEALTH

Kristina Y. Risley, DrPH, CPCC, is an Executive and Leadership Coach with Kris Risley Coaching. She has served the public health field in this role since being certified with the Co-Active Coaching Institute in 2004. Dr. Risley earned her DrPH in Maternal and Child Health from the University of Alabama at Birmingham. She also has a Master's Degree in Developmental Psychology; she has a sincere interest in the intersection of human and public health workforce development. Dr. Risley was also a staff and faculty member at the University of Illinois Chicago (UIC) School of Public Health between 2000 and 2018. In these roles, she focused on leadership development of the public health workforce. She worked closely with cross-sector partners to bring a leadership lens to the development of public health practitioners in the early 2000s. She continued this work as a faculty member with the UIC SPH Doctorate in Public Health Leadership Program. In this capacity, she taught a course on personal leadership development for public health practitioners committed to developing skills in systems change leadership. Dr. Risley brings an unapologetic heart to her work with public health professionals and it is this authentic expression that inspires those she works with to be more, do more, and to have greater meaning and impact in their work and more fulfillment in their lives.

Christina R. Welter, DrPH, MPH, is a nationally recognized policy practitioner, visionary leader, and practice-based researcher committed to helping organizations and communities co-create equity-centered systems change. She is a Clinical Assistant Professor in the Health Policy and Administration Division at the University of Illinois Chicago (UIC) School of Public Health where she also serves as the Director of the Doctorate in Public Health Leadership Program and the Associate Director of the Policy, Practice, and Prevention Research Center. Dr. Welter's scholarship focuses on mixed-method participatory action research and evaluation approaches to understand and address the structural determinants of health; facilitate learning, leadership development, and power building for structural change; and drive policy and systems change toward racial and economic justice. Dr. Welter oversees multiple applied research initiatives where she has catalyzed several award-winning cross-sectoral leadership collaboratives, co-designed novel capacity building initiatives, and built or translated evidence to foster policy adoption and implementation. Dr. Welter regularly provides technical assistance and serves in advisory capacities to facilitate strategic and transformative change. She proudly served as one of the Deputy Incident Commanders for the Illinois Department of Public Health's COVID-19 response during the Spring of 2020, helping the state to expand its strategic management, data systems, and policy response approaches. Prior to coming to UIC, Dr. Welter served as the Deputy Director at the Cook County Department of Public Health. Dr. Welter received her Doctorate in Public Health Leadership from the UIC School of Public Health and her Master's Degree in Public Health from the University of Michigan in Health Education and Health Behavior.

Grace Castillo, MPH, is a public health practitioner and health writer. She is particularly interested in public health infrastructure, science communication, and non communicable diseases. She is a Program Associate at the de Beaumont Foundation, where she focuses on project management for book publications. She has also volunteered with the Virginia Medical Reserve Corps. Previously, Ms. Castillo worked for the Equity Research and Innovation Center (ERIC) as a student research intern. While at ERIC, she supported a manuscript project documenting a collaborative steering committee's history. She also contributed to a draft guide for researchers interested in beginning community-based participatory research (CBPR). Ms. Castillo graduated from the Yale School of Public Health's Chronic Disease Epidemiology Department with a Certificate in Regulatory Affairs. While completing her Master of Public Health, Grace interned with the Patient-Centered Outcomes Research Institute (PCORI), where she worked with the Research Infrastructure team. She earned her BA in English from Yale University.

Brian C. Castrucci, DrPH, MA, is the President and Chief Executive Officer at the de Beaumont Foundation. Throughout his career, Brian has been a disruptor, instigator, and fierce advocate for the public's health. In the past 7 years, he has helped build the Foundation into a leading voice in health philanthropy and public health practice. He is an award-winning epidemiologist with 10 years of experience working in state and local governmental health agencies. He has authored more than 70 peer-reviewed journal articles, editorials, and book chapters and has shared his unique brand of practice-based thought leadership in blog posts and podcasts on several platforms, including *The Huffington Post, Governing,* Primary Care Progress Notes, KevinMD .com, Healthcare Leadership Blog at HCLDR.org, ASTHO's StatePublicHealth.org, and Health Affairs Blog.

LEADING SYSTEMS CHANGE IN PUBLIC HEALTH

A Field Guide for Practitioners

Kristina Y. Risley, DrPH, CPCC

Christina R. Welter, DrPH, MPH

Grace Castillo, MPH

Brian C. Castrucci, DrPH, MA

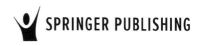

Springer Publishing Company, LLC
11 West 42nd Street, New York, NY 10036
www.springerpub.com

connect.springerpub.com/
Acquisitions Editor: David D'Addona
Compositor: S4Carlisle Publishing Services

ISBN: 978-0-8261-4508-6
ebook ISBN: 978-0-8261-4509-3
DOI: 10.1891/9780826145093

21 22 23 24 25 / 5 4 3 2 1

The author and the publisher of this Work have made every effort to use sources believed to be reliable to provide information that is accurate and compatible with the standards generally accepted at the time of publication. The author and publisher shall not be liable for any special, consequential, or exemplary damages resulting, in whole or in part, from the readers' use of, or reliance on, the information contained in this book. The publisher has no responsibility for the persistence or accuracy of URLs for external or third-party Internet websites referred to in this publication and does not guarantee that any content on such websites is, or will remain, accurate or appropriate.

Library of Congress Cataloging-in-Publication Data

Names: Risley, Kristina Y., author. | Welter, Christina R., author. |
  Castillo, Grace, author. | Castrucci, Brian C., author.
Title: Leading systems change in public health : a field guide for
  practitioners / [edited by] Kristina Y. Risley, Christina R. Welter,
  Grace Castillo, Brian C. Castrucci.
Identifiers: LCCN 2021038278 (print) | LCCN 2021038279 (ebook) | ISBN
  9780826145086 (cloth) | ISBN 9780826145093 (ebook)
Subjects: MESH: Public Health Administration—methods | Organizational
  Innovation | Leadership
Classification: LCC RA971 (print) | LCC RA971 (ebook) | NLM WA 525 | DDC
  362.1068–dc23
LC record available at https://lccn.loc.gov/2021038278
LC ebook record available at https://lccn.loc.gov/2021038279

Contact sales@springerpub.com to receive discount rates on bulk purchases.

Publisher's Note: New and used products purchased from third-party sellers are not guaranteed for quality, authenticity, or access to any included digital components

Printed in the United States of America.

This book is dedicated to public health practitioners:
You have dedicated your lives to public service.
You are committed to health, racial, and social justice.
We especially acknowledge your hard work during COVID-19
and your commitment to take a stand for racism as a critical public
health challenge that we can overcome.

Contents

Contributors

Millka Baetcke, MPH, MsMOB
Senior Managing Consultant
Integrated Solutions
Chicago, Illinois

Gina Massuda Barnett, MPH
Deputy Director
Public Health Programs
Cook County Department of Public Health
Forest Park, Illinois

Renée Branch Canady, PhD, MPA
CEO
Michigan Public Health Institute
Okemos, Michigan

Grace Castillo, MPH
Program Associate
de Beaumont Foundation
Bethesda, Maryland

Brian C. Castrucci, DrPH, MA
President and Chief Executive Officer
de Beaumont Foundation
Bethesda, Maryland

Dorothy Cilenti, DrPH, MPH, MSW
Associate Professor
Department of Maternal and Child Health
Gillings School of Global Public Health
The University of North Carolina at Chapel Hill
Chapel Hill, North Carolina

Samantha Cinnick, MPH, CHES, CPH
Program Officer
de Beaumont Foundation
Bethesda, Maryland

Ray Dlugolecki, MPH
Assistant Director of Public Health
Jackson County Health Department
Independence, Missouri

Lili Farhang, MPH
Co-Director
Human Impact Partners
Oakland, California

Lacy Fehrenbach, MPH, CPH
Deputy Secretary, COVID-19 Response
Washington State Department of Health
Olympia, Washington

W. Oscar Fleming, DrPH
Implementation Scientist
National Implementation Research Network
Clinical Assistant Professor
Department of Maternal and Child Health
Gillings School of Global Public Health
The University of North Carolina at Chapel Hill
Chapel Hill, North Carolina

Gillian Gawne-Mittlestaedt, DrPHc, MPA
Director
Partnership for Air Matters
Seattle, Washington

Solange Gould, DrPH, MPH
Co-Director
Human Impact Partners
Oakland, California

Kristen Hassmiller Lich, PhD
Associate Professor
Department of Health Policy and Management
Faculty Member
Executive Doctoral Program in Health Leadership
Gillings School of Global Public Health
University of North Carolina at Chapel Hill
Chapel Hill, North Carolina

Jeannine Herrick, MPH
Founder
Jeannine Herrick Leadership Coaching and Consulting
Adjunct Faculty
Public Health Leadership
Gillings School of Global Public Health
University of North Carolina at Chapel Hill
Chapel Hill, North Carolina

Cynthia D. Lamberth, PhDc, MPH, CPH
Executive Director
Kentucky Population Health Institute
Frankfort, Kentucky

Patricia Moten Marshall, MHA
President
SynerChange Chicago
Chicago, Illinois

Mary F. Morten, BA
President
Morten Group, LLC
Chicago, Illinois

Amy Mullenix, MSPH, MSW
Senior Collaboration Manager
Maternal Health Learning & Innovation Center
National MCH Workforce Development Center
Department of Maternal and Child Health
Gillings School of Global Public Health
The University of North Carolina at Chapel Hill
Chapel Hill, North Carolina

Golda Philip, JD, MPH
Senior Advisor for Equity
Maternal and Child Health Bureau
Health Resources Services Administration
U.S. Department of Health and Human Services
Rockville, Maryland

Eve C. Pinsker, PhD
Clinical Assistant Professor
Department of Community Health Sciences
Core Faculty Member
Doctorate in Public Health Leadership
School of Public Health
University of Illinois Chicago
Chicago, Illinois

Geneva Porter, MPH
Project Director
Morten Group, LLC
Chicago, Illinois

Kristina Y. Risley, DrPH, CPCC
Senior Advisor
de Beaumont Foundation
Executive and Leadership Coach
Kris Risley Coaching
Chicago, Illinois

Karen Trierweiler, MS, CNM (Retired)
Founding Partner
Total Population Health, LLC
Denver, Colorado

Jonathan Webb, MPH, MBA
CEO
Association of Women's Health
Obstetric and Neonatal Nurses
Washington, DC

Rebecca Wells, MHSA, PhD
Professor
Department of Management, Policy, and Community Health
The University of Texas School of Public Health
Houston, Texas

Christina R. Welter, DrPH, MPH
Director
DrPH in Leadership
Associate Director
Policy, Practice, and Prevention Research Center
Clinical Assistant Professor
Department of Health Policy and Administration
School of Public Health
University of Illinois Chicago
Chicago, Illinois

Preface

The goal of this book is to provide a framework for how to develop a strategic public health workforce that is capable of addressing complex challenges to achieve health justice and racial and social equity. Over the decades, there has been a growing focus on the evolving learning and development needs of those of us working in the field of public health. Broadly speaking, we are technical experts in how to improve the public's health. However, because of the increasingly complex world in which we live, highlighted most recently by coronavirus disease 2019 (COVID-19) and unrest due to the racial, health, and social inequities that continue to exist in our country, we must expand our skills to include those necessary to lead systems change.

This book aims to:

- Provide a common language for practitioners to discuss systems thinking and leading systems change
- Offer key principles for systems change leadership
- Deliver a framework for individuals and organizations who want to lead systems change
- Offer public health examples and practical exercises, practices, and tools to engage in leading systems change

Public health practitioners have a passion to improve population health and health equity. This work requires the will and capacity to lead cross-sector efforts to achieve the outcomes we know are possible. If we are to achieve these outcomes, a focus on systems change leadership and learning is needed now more than ever. These skills combined with our technical skills present a unique opportunity to transform our society into one that takes a stand for the evolution of our country—a country that places equity squarely in the heart of our work and who we are as a nation.

In this book, renowned systems change leaders and practitioners in public health share their expertise, experiences, and tools for leading across and within the critical levels of systems change. Authors include the co-directors of Human Impact Partners, Lili Farhang and Solange Gould; leaders in the National Maternal and Child Health Workforce Development Center, Dorothy Cilenti, Amy Mullenix, Kristen Hassmiller

Lich, Oscar Fleming, Rebecca Wells, Karen Trierweiler, and Jeannine Herrick; organizational change experts including Patricia Moten Marshall, Mary Morten, Geneva Porter, and Renée Branch Canady; and other local, state, and national public health leaders who are committed to leading change in our systems, including Gina Massuda Barnett, Milka Baetcke, Grace Castillo, Brian Castrucci, Sam Cinnick, Ray Dlugolecki, Lacey Fehrenbach, Cynthia Lamberth, Gillian Mittelstaedt, Golda Phillip, Eve Pinsker, Kristina Risley, Jonathan Webb, and Christina Welter.

These authors demystify what it means to lead systems change, and they provide the tools necessary to be systems change leaders. Together, they offer a framework for the ways in which individuals and organizations can achieve public health improvements by leading systems change across and within critical levels. When it comes to leading systems change, there is no wrong entry point. We can begin this work at the individual level—who am I as a public health leader and what do I or will I stand for? We can also begin this work with the teams on which we work. Some may choose to begin at the organizational level and still others may begin this work with the communities they serve. This book is designed to meet you where you are, so jump in where it makes the most sense to you.

Leading systems change in public health is an evolving science and practice. Systems thinking by its nature facilitates sharing different perspectives and different approaches about how to undertake this important work. As such, authors in this book may differ on how to frame, where to start, and how to undertake systems change. Further, their perspectives on a topic may transform with new practice-based experiences and as our understanding of systems change evolves over time. Author approaches to systems change may or may not be like how you envision systems change. We are all learning and growing in similar and different ways when it comes to systems change work. We are developing greater individual and collective awareness around the important issues and strategies addressed in this book. As such, it is necessary to bring deep humility and a willingness to change and grow with each small and large step forward. For example, given ongoing efforts to address racism in this country, there are current discussions about the use of uppercase and lowercase letters to describe (white) race. For different philosophical reasons, some authors use lowercase "w" when referring to white race; others use uppercase "W" to refer to White race. To highlight the importance of staying in the conversation and respecting diverse viewpoints, this book uses uppercase letters to describe all races except when those engaged utilize a different practice. The editors and publishers of this book felt it important to respect all sides of this issue especially in this time when solutions are not clear-cut. When this is the case, it is noted in the chapter.

Change is inevitable, and how you lead through it is up to you. The COVID-19 pandemic along with the racial uprisings throughout our nation to take a stand for an equitable nation for all will bring necessary change in our country and how we engage in public health practice. There are already new and significant federal investments being made to improve the public health workforce. These investments alone will not bring change. Change is deliberate. While the resources may increase, we need the skills to shape our public health practice in the future.

It is our sincere hope that you will find this book to be a useful and practical tool for your own development and the development of the workforce within your agencies and organizations. We hope that it can serve as a tool to set the conversation around what it means to lead systems change and that it can be used to guide conversations about the importance of supporting the lifelong growth, learning, and development of the workforce. This book is meant to be a starting point and not the destination. We hope that it is useful and that you share your lessons learned about what works, what does not work, what is and is not clear, and what can further our knowledge of leading change.

We welcome you to visit our webpage for the book at debeaumont.org/books/leading-systems-change where you may find additional resources. Please feel free to share with us your feedback, as we would love to hear from you!

Kristina Y. Risley
Christina R. Welter
Grace Castillo
Brian C. Castrucci

The de Beaumont Foundation: Bold Solutions for Healthier Communities

Founded in 1998, the de Beaumont Foundation advances policy, builds partnerships, and strengthens public health to create communities where people can achieve their best possible health. To that end, the de Beaumont Foundation creates and invests in bold solutions that improve the health of communities across the entire country.

Our focus on policy seeks to ensure that current and future generations can benefit from changes enacted by today's leaders; our work on partnerships brings unlikely allies together so that leaders can achieve the shared goals of creating healthier communities; and our emphasis on people helps us create practical solutions that strengthen the public health system and workforce so that professionals are equipped to make their communities healthier.

The de Beaumont Foundation's initiatives include CityHealth, the BUILD Health Challenge, the Public Health Workforce Interests and Needs Survey (PHWINS), Public Health Reaching Across Sectors (PHRASES), 40 Under 40 in Public Health, the Big Cities Health Coalition (BCHC), the Building Expertise in Administration and Management (BEAM) certificate course, the National Consortium for Public Health Workforce Development, and numerous publications by the field, for the field. For more information, please visit https://debeaumont.org/.

Acknowledgments

The publication of this book took the efforts of far more people than just the editors. We would like to thank the book's Advisory Group; they provided early and ongoing input into our thinking and helped shape the topics we chose to address. Members included Patricia Moten Marshall, President of SynerChange Chicago; Lili Farhang, Co-Executive Director of the Human Impact Partners in Oakland, CA; Jonathan Webb, CEO of the Association of Women's Health, Obstetric and Neonatal Nurses; Jeannine Herrick, Founder, Jeannine Herrick Leadership Coaching and Consulting; and Samantha Cinnick, Program Officer, de Beaumont Foundation. This group convened just as the COVID-19 pandemic began; they stayed the course. Their wisdom, expertise, and enthusiasm brought this book alive. The process of creating this book together with them was rewarding because of the depth and breadth they brought to our discussions.

Thank you also to our colleagues at Springer Publishing Company, who have been wonderful partners. From the first day we talked with David D'Addona, Senior Editor, at the American Public Health Association (APHA) conference in Philadelphia in 2019, we have been compellingly and firmly led by his calm and clear demeanor and confident vision about the importance of this content. Jaclyn Shultz, Associate Editor of Health Sciences, has led a beautiful process to keep us moving forward daily. When things felt challenging, she found an easy way forward.

We would also like to acknowledge the authors. In the middle of the pandemic, they agreed to take on this additional, unanticipated writing project and our ambitious timeline for completion. They graciously said yes to our call to provide their expertise about how to lead systems change in public health just as their systems and our world was changing in unknown and unpredictable ways; they too stayed the course. Each generously shared their unique perspective, expertise, experience, and wisdom beautifully on the written page. We are grateful for their willingness to step into the unknown with us and partner together to bring this book to the field. We are excited to share their expertise with you.

We also want to acknowledge the leaders and mentors who have come before us as well as those of you currently working in the field of public health. We share your fierce loyalty to the field and to efforts that improve the public's health. Your collective dedication to systems change, including addressing the root causes of the inequities in our nation, captures the sense of selfless commitment among public health practitioners that inspires us to continue these efforts. We see all of you as thought partners who have helped to shape this work; this book is infused with your voices. We acknowledge and are grateful for the education, support, and encouragement we have and continue to receive from all of you.

Each of the editors has been shaped by mentors who have guided us through our professional careers. Drs. Welter and Risley would like to especially acknowledge and thank Drs. Patrick Lenihan and Lou Rowitz. Drs. Lenihan and Rowitz have spent decades influencing the field of public health, mentoring and training public health practitioners to critically examine public health challenges in ways that highlight the adaptive versus technical elements, approach situations from the leadership versus management lens, and to develop novel and strategic approaches to facilitate systems change in enduring ways. Their ideas and coaching influenced our thinking and the direction of this field guide. Dr. Risley would also like to acknowledge Dr. Arden Handler who modeled courage and boldness and taking a stand for challenging the status quo. Dr. Welter would like to acknowledge Dr. Jill Korbin and Susan Troia for their endless encouragement and mentorship. Dr. Castrucci would like to acknowledge Ms. Nancy Kaufman who was a driver of change throughout her career in public health and philanthropy and a personal mentor for more than 20 years. Ms. Kaufman passed away in May 2021. This book is a testament to her continued influence. Ms. Castillo would like to acknowledge the entire staff at ERIC and all advisors, teachers, supervisors, and mentors over the years.

Finally, this work would not have been possible without the support of Dr. James B. Sprague and the de Beaumont Foundation Board of Directors, and, as always, thank you, Pete.

Introduction: Inspired by the Past, Empowering the Future

As you begin your use of this field guide on leading systems change it is important to take a quick glance at the history of public health leadership development to examine what we might build on from those programs and efforts and how we might empower and build more effectiveness, sustainability, and equity into our current efforts.

Public health has a long history of preventing disease through assessment, policy, and assurance. "John Snow, the father of epidemiology, removed the handle from the broad street pump and, with this single act of leadership, proved that contaminated water indeed spread cholera."[1] This story illustrates the decisive action often required of public health leaders and is an early example of using systems thinking to understand root causes. In the end, the solution to this problem was simple; however, it required working with residents and council members to identify the problem. Trained epidemiologists learn to ask, "Where is the pump handle on this challenge?"[2] Like Snow, they are looking for the one action or series of actions that can save lives and reduce health inequities.

Today's challenges are quite complex. They require systems thinking, yes, but the solutions are many; some solutions are simple and easily result in our desired outcomes whereas others are complicated and, when addressed, may produce unintended consequences. Complex problems require diverse cross-sector stakeholders and leadership across stakeholders to achieve intended and sustainable results. The coronavirus disease 2019 (COVID-19) pandemic is an example of a complex problem. The solutions were many; some simple, some complicated. Much of the response, however, required intricate coordination, alignment, and collaboration with quite an extensive and diverse set of stakeholders. The pandemic exposed the impact of not having a systems thinking skillset that leads to systems change leadership. This skillset is necessary to swiftly facilitate collective thought and decisive action. Without it, we continue to address complex problems as if they are simple or even complicated problems. As a result, the solutions we identify, at best, only partially solve a problem, and at worst, they create more complex problems than where we started.

Throughout history, decisive leaders' actions have encouraged others by example. Three examples of beautiful historic actions include Mary Breckenridge's establishment of neonatal and childhood medical care systems serving rural Kentucky, Mary Mahoney demanding greater equality for people of color as the first African American licensed nurse, and Grace Abbott's resolve to improve the right of immigrants, advancing child welfare, and regulating child labor. Although their process may not be evident or explicit, these women were inspirational leaders who serve as models for today's public health leaders about what can be achieved by focusing on the passion and will to make changes. They remind us of the need to focus on systems change leadership by engaging with diverse partners. They were engaging in systems change work even before they had the training and development to support them. Today more than ever, we need an explicit focus on providing development of systems change leaders. But, first, let us take a historical look at the past to remember our journey toward the development of systems change leaders and be inspired and empowered to impact the future of systems change driven by the will of leaders and the communities they serve.

COMPETENCY-BASED LEADER DEVELOPMENT

Explicit calls for leadership and development of those who serve the public were highlighted in both the 1988[3] and 2002[4] Institute of Medicine reports focused on public health. The identification of those gaps laid the groundwork for several decades of funding at the federal level from the Centers for Disease Control and Prevention (CDC) and the Health Resources and Services Administration (HRSA). Numerous local, state, and national foundations also funded initiatives seeking to improve the public health system by developing the individuals that lead governmental, private, and non profit health focused organizations. This created a several decades–long investment in competency-based public health[5] leadership development and created National, Regional and State Public Health Leadership Institutes (PHLI) and profession-specific leadership institutes, including Nursing, Environmental, Maternal and Child Health, Health Educators, Epidemiologists, and Laboratorians.

These programs introduced systems thinking, utilized action learning and case study methods, focused on teamwork, and addressed specific competencies unique to public health leaders developed by the National Leadership Development Network (NLN) workgroup.[6] As challenges to public health emerged, including communicable outbreaks, drug misuse, increases in chronic disease, persistent health inequities, and terrorism, the leadership training responded with new competency-based trainings.[7] The attacks of 9/11 profoundly affected leadership development as programs pivoted to provide crisis leadership and crisis communication-focused competency development.

The leadership programs utilized a systems approach to leadership that called for synthesized wisdom (knowledge with application), creativity, and intelligence, translated into strategic evidence-based programs and policies driven by the will of the community.[1] This strategic approach allowed for both creative and systems thinking and emphasized the need for community involvement and will to enact changes. However, this approach was still widely focused on the individual leader rather than the collective team-based, community-focused efforts necessary to address complex and "wicked"[8,9] problems.

TRANSITION TO A NEW COLLECTIVE VIEW OF LEADERSHIP

As the leadership development programs responded to novel problems and increased evidence became available through data, the pedagogy focus included team-based, action learning approaches at the national level[10] as well as many regional and state-based programs. This change allowed for more inclusive and generative conversations to tackle problems including mental health, drug misuse, and the opioid crisis. Some programs also facilitated learners self-forming into teams, again seeking to solve real-world problems by bringing many diverse voices to the table. However, these efforts, although team-based, continued to be primarily focused on technical solutions versus adaptive solutions.

The results of these team-based, community-focused efforts were shared and replicated in many locations. A recognition program named after one of the early and long-standing champions of leadership development at the CDC, Tom Balderson,[11] provided an opportunity for teams to compete with others based on the impact of the project, and the competition's, results in the winning teams presented at APHA each year.

Evaluation of the efforts of the National Leadership Programs solidified efficacy of team action learning format both as perceived by the participants and the agencies utilizing the projects.[12] The ability to network with other leaders on mutual problem-solving and community-based interventions was also highly valued by participants.

These findings supported the continued efforts and creation of communities of practice,[13] the Public Health Leadership Society (alumni of the programs) and Code of Public Health Ethics,[14] and the National Leadership Development Network (NLN).[15] The NLN, initially comprised of all the CDC leadership institute grantees, expanded to include all those working in the public sector leadership space, adding important focus on diverse leadership programming. The NLN group (no longer active) collectively created a conceptual model for leadership development,[6] Leadership Competency Framework in PH Leadership.[6] They also created specific tools, including a PH Leadership 360 assessment, Crisis Leadership online modules, and the previously mentioned Tom Balderson Awards. Today, several state or regional leadership institutes, still operate including the National Leadership Academy for the Public's Health,[10] bringing together teams of leaders from multiple sectors who actively engage their communities to improve population health and achieve health equity.

WHAT WE LEARNED

The focus on public health leadership in the last few decades of the 20th century also sharpened the differences between public health and other leaders. Public sector work requires problem-solving and decision-making that impacts the public good. In public health, there is a commitment to racial and social justice that ideally will translate into health equity. Moore has argued that the challenge behind public sector work is the need to create public value for the work.[16] If constituencies do not see the value or if political priorities do not rank the work as high priority, the public health leader struggles. We also learned that year-long programs, while costly when conducted in-person, offer a unique time period to work on real problems in a team, creating valuable work products and meaningful networking. The ability of curriculum developers to engage in collective development, research, and publications is also of note.

We also found that simple short-term learning, including book clubs; blog posts, alumni networks; social media groups; and informal facilitation of networking, coaching, and mentoring helped keep the leaders invigorated and supported in using their new skills.

The flexibility to rebrand around systems leadership, which includes understanding the root causes of complex problems like pandemics, is critical. Community-based multisectoral work produces lasting change and creates actions and stories to support sustainably.

EMPOWERING THE FUTURE

The past decade brought forth new calls to action for leadership development and responses utilizing collective approaches with heart-centered community dialogue that demand listening to the voices of all people. It also called for greater attention to the community conditions, social determinants of health, that create health including a prominent focus on racism as a public health problem that must be addressed with a wide range of stakeholders at a systems level if we are to achieve health equity.

The need for systems change leadership is supported by the iterative nature of developing leaders that emerged by responding to current challenges and changes in the public health workforce.[17] The need to address structural inequities within our organizations, racism, and the pandemic response are opportunities to learn and codify our approaches even more. Successful change occurs by bringing together diverse, traditional, and non traditional stakeholders to identify root causes of complex problems and align around common agendas to improve community health.

Individual leaders still need to develop as leaders, commit to strong interpersonal relationships as well as team development (internal and cross-sector teams), and establish strong relationships with community partners who are experts in improving their communities. Further, the COVID-19 pandemic has once again emphasized the need for strong and consistent communication from leaders utilizing crisis and risk communication best practices.

Our history and efforts over the past three decades created many initiatives culminating in community-empowered leaders making a difference in the health of their communities. Many of these stories are provided within this book to celebrate accomplishments and spur others into action. Much of this work uses research, evidence, and dissemination approaches to achieve health equity. Applying lessons from the past will include expanding the focus on individual development, including self-awareness, authentic self-expression, empathy, and compassion, alongside team-focused leadership development through action learning applied to multisectoral teams. The use of evidence-based frameworks, models, and principles including the Learning Agenda Toolkit[18] will assist in the development of an adaptive workforce through life-long learning and health equity.

WHY SYSTEMS LEADERSHIP, WHY NOW?

As the complexity of public health increased, a systems perspective was employed that creates initiatives that are community-based and help the agency better relate to internal and external stakeholders. Today we recognize leaders are not only the collective designers of the creative process, but they are also the standard bearers for the system that is strengthened through the work of the collective will. The role of the leader is not only to guide and promote the creative and systemic process but to commit and support the outcomes.

The most pressing topic within this field book is the increase in focus on equity, power, privilege, and racial and social justice. We have begun to challenge the individual leadership narrative focused on meritocracy and individual achievement by increasing our focus on health and racial equity. Without equity at the center of all leadership development and work, we risk continuing to contribute to structural effects. We need systems change and leaders equipped to enact those changes. What systems change looks like in our organizations and communities is explored in detail in this field book. How we orchestrate the WILL to create a vibrant, responsive, admired public health system, workforce, and leaders focused on health equity is our greatest challenge! I leave you with the challenge to lean into that WILL.

When President John F. Kennedy asked Dr. Wernher von Braun what it would take to build a rocket that could carry a man to the moon and bring him back safely to the Earth, von Braun answered him in five words, "The will to do it."

The will to do it is "something that wakes you up in the morning and gets you excited about it, or something that makes you so angry, you know you have to do something about it," in the words of Stacey Abrams.

What would it take to create a vibrant, responsive, admired public health system, workforce, and leaders that ensure equitable and optimal health for all people and communities? The will to do it.

Do public health leaders wake up each morning so excited about the work, determined to do something about it?

Cynthia D. Lamberth, PhDc, MPH, CPH
Executive Director
Kentucky Population Health Institute
Frankfort, Kentucky

REFERENCES

1. Lamberth CD, Rowitz L. Leadership chapter. In: Scutchfield FD, Keck CW, eds. *Principles of Public Health Practice* 3rd ed. Delmar Cengage Learning; 2009.
2. Snow J. *On the Mode of Communication of Cholera*. John Churchil; 1855.
3. Institute of Medicine. *The Future of Public Health*. The National Academies Press; 1988. doi:10.17226/1091.
4. Gebbie K, Rosenstock L, Hernandez, LM (Eds.). *Institute of Medicine (US) Committee on educating public health professionals for the 21st century*. National Academies Press (US); 2003.
5. *Core Competencies for Public Health Professionals*. Council on Linkages Between Academia and Public Health Practice; 2021.
6. Wright K, Rowitz L, Merkle A, Reid, WM, Robinson G, Herzog B, Weber D, Carmichael D, Balderson TR, Baker E. Competency development in public health leadership. *American Journal of Public Health*. 2000;90 90(8) 1202–1207. doi:10.2105/ajph.90.8.1202.
7. Hawley SR, St. Romain T, Orr SA, Molgaard CA, Kabler BS. Competency-based impact of a statewide public health leadership training program. *Health Promotion Practice*. 2000;12(2): 202–208. doi:10.1177/1524839909349163.
8. Conklin J. *Dialogue Mapping: Building Shared Understanding of Wicked Problems*. John Wiley & Sons; 2005.
9. Conklin J. *Wicked Problems and Social Complexity*. CogNexus Institute; 2006, 11.
10. Helping local, state, and national leaders to address the most pressing challenges in public health. Center for Health Leadership & Practice website. https://healthleadership.org/programs/nlaph.
11. Blackford A. National award recognizes public health training program project to improve emergency response. University of Kentucky UKnow; October 2, 2011. https://uknow.uky.edu/professional-news/national-award-recognizes-public-health-training-program-project-improve-emergency.
12. Umble K, Steffen D, Porter J, Miller D, Hummer-McLaughlin K, Lowman A, Zelt S. The National Public Health Leadership Institute: Evaluation of a team-based approach to developing collaborative public health leaders. *American Journal of Public Health*. 2005;92(4):641–644. doi:10.2105/AJPH.2004.047993.
13. Wheatley M. *Supporting Pioneering Leaders as Communities of Practice: How to Rapidly Develop New Leaders in Great Numbers*. The Berkana Institute; 2002.
14. Thomas JC, Sage M, Dillenberg J, Guillory VJ. A code of ethics for public health. *American Journal of Public Health*. 2002;92(7):1057–1059. doi:10.2105/ajph.92.7.1057.
15. National Public Health Leadership Development Network website (no longer online).
16. Moore MH. *Creating Public Value: Strategic Management in Government*. Harvard University Press; 1995.
17. Gould E, Castrucci B, Bogaert K, Sellers K, Leider J. Changes in the state governmental public health workforce: 2014–2017. *Journal of Public Health Management & Practice*. 2019;25(Suppl. 2):S58–S66. doi:10.1097/PHH.0000000000000933.
18. Public Health Learning Agenda. http://www.publichealthlearningagenda.org/. Accessed April 23, 2021.

Framing Systems Change

1

The Time Is Now for Leading Systems Change in Public Health Practice

Eve C. Pinsker, Christina R. Welter, and Kristina Y. Risley

INTRODUCTION

For those of us working in public health, especially during the challenges and destabilization of coronavirus disease 2019 (COVID-19) and racial unrest, it is clearer than ever that we need new skills for addressing increasingly complex problems. We must continue with the usual activities of public health—the work we were trained to do to ensure a healthy populace—while we examine what holds us back from achieving the public health outcomes we all desire. Why do we not see the improvements in public health that we know are possible?

This book addresses that question and provides a framework and process for addressing complex challenges that speak to long-standing and seemingly intractable problems within our outdated systems and structures. It provides the evidence and tools you need to build a strong systems change leadership approach to your work—whether you are new to your career or are a seasoned public health professional. To be systems change leaders and public health strategists, we must develop this new skill set at multiple levels: our individual leadership contribution to public health, regardless of title; our interpersonal relationships as a leadership tool; our organizations as public health leaders or public health strategists; and our leadership on internal, external, and cross-sector teams and with the communities we serve—community members and community stakeholders (education, housing, transportation, business, for example). Most important, we need to develop these skills using an equity lens that allows us to build capacity in health equity and racial and social justice work both within and outside our organizations.

First, we define systems thinking and systems change leadership in public health practice and then explain why we wrote the book, key principles of systems change leadership, and useful systems change resources. We also discuss the intended audience for the book. Next, we provide an overview of how the book is organized, including what you can expect across chapters, and suggestions about how to use the book. Last, we reflect on these chapters and systems change leadership in the context of the environment we are in as the book goes into production. We wrote this chapter as the final component of compiling this book, which started around the time COVID-19 was declared a pandemic in March 2020. We hope that you appreciate these materials as a work in progress; we know that these ideas and tools will evolve as those of us in the field take hold of them and make them our own.

SYSTEMS THINKING AND SYSTEMS CHANGE LEADERSHIP IN PUBLIC HEALTH PRACTICE

Public health practitioners bring a wealth of technical training—in epidemiology and the spread of infectious diseases, in the multiple causes of chronic disease, in the ways that environmental toxins can affect human health, in the assessment of public and private resources needed to support healthy communities, and much more—to their work in the world. As technical training progresses, it tends to follow the path of specialization. In short, practitioners learn more about less. Reduction accompanies specialization, simplifying complex contexts into a few variables that can be more easily manipulated in the service of explanation and prediction.

While this knowledge has made valuable contributions to community health and well-being, predictions that are successful in controlled conditions often fail when tested in the context of real-world communities and complex human lives. Knowledge that can be applied to produce practical solutions to our problems must successfully grapple with webs of material resources, politics, and organizational procedures. Applicable knowledge also must contend with the diverse and often conflicting perspectives of community members and power brokers as well as scientists. Fortunately, the 20th century saw the rise of scientific paradigms that countered reductionist visions with more holistic approaches to knowledge, highlighting complex interactions and directing attention to diverse contexts. Frameworks and models for systems theory and systems science developed within and across multiple disciplines. Public health has applied systems science tools, including network analysis and causal loop modeling, to disparate topics such as tobacco coalitions and the increase in obesity and diabetes (see note).[1-3]

Note: "Systems thinking" is not one unified discipline or field. In the 20th century and continuing into the 21st, there have been many lines of theory development and practice based in different disciplines and conversations between them that shared the goal of understanding and practically engaging with complex patterns of connection and wholes that are more than the sum of their parts, while maintaining scientific empiricism and analytical rigor but going beyond reductionist science or social science paradigms that isolate variables and ignore context. For a useful synthesis of how these "systems lineages" from thinkers rooted in biology, anthropology, mathematics, engineering, psychology, etc., have resulted in multiple contemporary schools of systems

Practitioners have extended these new ways of thinking beyond theory and science to new paradigms for approaching practical problems that go beyond technical knowledge to everyday action in the world. Just as those in business and family therapy have applied "systems thinking" within their fields, so too can public health practitioners apply its methods to leading change. Moreover, its practice can be deeply democratic. Systems thinking encourages us to ask about the underlying causes of ill-being that we experience, about how our habitual assumptions and values are part of the challenges we face, and about where there are small openings we can use to leverage greater change. Discussions about these types of questions can and should include community members without technical training as well as practitioners from other sectors and disciplines. We hope that this book will help public health practitioners and emerging leaders have such conversations productively and, in collaboration with diverse partners, build on them with action.

Building Partnerships to Address Complex Challenges

Public health leaders must work collaboratively to address complex challenges like the roots of health inequity, shifting the social determinants of health to improve health and well-being, and mitigation and adaptation to climate change and its effects on health. To move the needle on these complex problems, public health leaders must interact with multiple levels and circles of others, including legislators; "ordinary" citizens and community members; and practitioners from other sectors, such as education or regional planning. We need to examine and rethink our circles of influence, which comprise with whom we interact and how. Complex problems require us to engage and collaborate with traditional partners and organizations in new ways; they also require us to collaborate or coordinate with new partners. Complex problems require coordinated efforts across a range of public and private partners as well as intricate collaborations, which require strategic practices that can and must be learned if we are to adapt to and shape a changing world.

Public health is inclined to lead collective partnerships to advance community priorities, and these partnerships often bring diverse stakeholders to the table. This inclination is not always built into the fabric of the work in other sectors, however. In addition, public health practitioners' inclination to lead partnerships does not always translate into possessing the skills to lead collaborative efforts. That next step requires identifying and then cultivating those skills.

---

practice, see R. Ison, *Systems Practice: How to Act: In Situations of Uncertainty and Complexity in a Climate Change World.* 2nd ed. Springer; 2017:30–36. For a description of multiple tools useful in social intervention work stemming from diverse systems thinking approaches, see Bob Williams and Richard Hummelbrunner. *Systems Concepts in Action: A Practitioner's Toolkit.* Stanford University Press; 2011. Public health scientists and practitioners in the United States have generally drawn from only a few of these systems lineages, emphasizing, for instance, causal loop analysis from systems dynamics as developed by Jay Forrester and applied (without Forrester's computer simulation modeling) to organizational development by Peter Senge, but see the special issue of the *American Journal of Public Health* from May 2006 that also draws from soft systems and critical systems heuristics approaches better known in the United Kingdom (G. Midgley. Systemic intervention for public health. *Am J Public Health.* 2006; 96:466–472).

The near future offers opportunities for public health practitioners and those who train emerging public health leaders. COVID-19 has heightened awareness among the public and policy makers of public health and its crucial worth. In response to the pandemic, the Biden administration announced a plan to invest over $7 billion to hire and train public health workers, including a new grant program to expand, train, and modernize our public health workforce. This workforce of the future will require a systems thinking skill set to lead collaborative and collective efforts to ensure that antiquated systems and structures are modernized. These actions will allow us to focus on the core of what public health has stood for and continues to stand for: population (versus individual) health; prevention; and the upstream factors affecting health and well-being, including health equity and racial and social justice.

WHY DID WE WRITE THIS BOOK?

Imagining Our Desired Future

We wrote this book to provide insight into the systems thinking skills needed to engage in systems change leadership and to provide our colleagues in public health with direction in how to cultivate these skills as we continue to learn and cultivate these skills in ourselves. This type of educational and professional development, leading to an improved capacity to engage in systems change leadership, will enable us to work toward a world in which all people are seen, valued, and have every opportunity for whole health.

Imagine a future where public health practitioners are scientists and systems change leaders who mobilize communities to achieve such a world. Imagine a future where systems are in place for public health practitioners at all levels of experience to engage in lifelong learning that emboldens them to initiate and support transformation of our systems, policies, processes, and practices to be more equitable, inclusive, and effective. Because public health practitioners genuinely have this worldview, it is a natural fit for them to lead the way toward realizing this vision. Imagine an adaptive and resilient workforce that has the internal and external resources to address complex change, emerging threats, and long-standing social and racial injustice. Imagine a world where we collectively acknowledge and face the consequences of the injustices of the past on the health of all in the present and move to redress those consequences and give all people the opportunity to live to their full potential for health and well-being.

Such a charge must be considered within the larger world context. This includes highlighting challenges such as transitioning from the industrial to the knowledge era, which requires workers with different skill sets than in the past. In the past, it was sufficient to have technical skills to address simple and even complicated problems. Today our complex problems require different skill sets for responding to that complexity. This includes adjusting to the speed of change—the exponential amount of change we face today compared with just a decade ago. With the arrival of COVID-19, our relationship with change began to evolve again—the virus introduced us to constant change at a time when we already were struggling to manage an accelerated pace of change. Compounding that, public health shares the demands placed on the private sector, in the United States and nations under austerity regimes, of doing more with less at a time when more and not less is needed.

The pandemic has highlighted the stress of the wicked, grave, global challenges specifically facing public health: Epidemics and other disasters occur with increasing frequency due to the foreseeable consequences of interlocking cycles of human population growth and unsustainable resource use coupled with persistent socioeconomic inequities within and between nations. These challenges call for changing behaviors as well as changing cultures, examining long-standing mindsets, and cultivating open-mindedness. These shifts are essential if we are to have any chance of dismantling entrenched systems and building new systems that help workforces and communities thrive. They also require that efforts be directed at developing a skillful workforce that can take on these challenges.

Systems change leadership—leading change not only in human behavior but in the underlying assumptions and consequent structures that drive behavior—is not for the faint of heart. It does, however, give us opportunities to modernize our organizational, economic, social, and political systems and to dismantle old and oppressive systems by developing relationships and co-creating with diverse partners. Systems change leadership provides opportunities to build new, equitable systems that help all people thrive and to create cultures where learning and evolving is the standard. Through a commitment to learning, we grow in our leadership, our approach to work, our ability to impact public health outcomes, and ultimately in our capacity to contribute to a sustainable world. Further, as part of systems change leadership, we hold ourselves accountable for what we say we will do, creating systems that have resources and policies in place to help sustain and evolve us over time. We seek and create openings to shift mindsets and imagine as well as create possibilities for new ways of distributing resources and supporting health for all.

Systems change leadership means that we focus on prevention rather than continue to deal with the fallout of the structures and procedures that we have inherited or created over time. To be systems change leaders, we need to be courageous; we must stretch toward upstream efforts and be bold in leading approaches that enable us—a broadly inclusive "us"—to collectively and strategically focus on health equity and racial justice.

Working Upstream to Challenge the Status Quo

Working at multiple levels—including personal, interpersonal—and organizational—and through diverse and cross-sector teams that include community members and other community stakeholders, we as systems change leaders are committed to being agents of change who challenge the status quo. We consider the larger system, engage in reflective and generative conversations, and move quickly from defining a problem to co-creating a shared vision of the future with diverse partners who reflect multiple perspectives and experiences of current challenges.[4] This work requires us to learn and practice working collaboratively and in coordination with diverse stakeholders. It also requires us as leaders to engage in lifelong learning and development at multiple levels. We must develop ourselves as leaders, learn to be good team members, engage in work that enables our organizations to be on the leading edge of public health change, and create with our communities. We must share a willingness to examine the positionality and power within our existing systems, organizations, and in ourselves. We must continue to hold a commitment to health equity, anti-racism, and social justice. This work requires us to examine entrenched assumptions, beliefs, and mental models that maintain the status quo at best and hold back humanity at worst. This work will enable us to build personal and shared visions that lead to creative and inspired public health innovations.

To this end, we must be willing to look at the complexity of our challenges, including the deep questioning necessary to identify root causes. This requires a dynamic and interactive process examining the internal and external factors driving a problem as well as a willingness to imagine a shared future. Then, we must be willing to face the tension between what is and what could be rather than passively accepting the status quo. We need to develop strategies for leading change inside the organizations we are part of as well as strategies for leading change externally, whether it be with local, regional, national, or global partners. That means being willing to share human and financial resources. Further, we must share decision-making power about how to allocate these resources toward a collaboratively envisioned, mutually desired future.

A commitment to becoming effective agents of systems change requires being comfortable with iterative cycles of reflecting, assessing, planning, acting, and learning. It requires engaging with people who have different perspectives and being willing to listen and truly hear and be curious about where another person is coming from and then finding common ground from which to align and move forward together. This includes both accountability for progress toward shared goals and a commitment to "fail forward," understanding that in a complex world we will not always hit our intended targets but will learn from our failures and recalibrate or re-evaluate our objectives.

Sustaining valued long-term goals may require change and evolution of the strategies we thought would get us there, as well as questioning and clarification of what it is that we want to sustain and what we want to change. This includes learning what we must change if we are to achieve an equitable, diverse, and just human society within a sustainable and diverse ecosystem. To succeed, we need to learn how to effectively reach out to multiple audiences, those who share our commitment to a collective investment in public health and health equity, and those who do not, and critically consider the consequences of how we frame and brand our efforts.

WHY READ THIS BOOK?

These chapters represent work in progress—the beginning of a journey to systems change leadership. They are designed for busy public health practitioners who want to quickly integrate systems change tools into their work. We believe the material presented here will help you gain clarity about the drivers of health and inequities, provide clear opportunities for systems change leadership at multiple levels, and serve as a resource so that more people in the public health workforce are ready to take a role in leading change. It will support development of individuals as systems change leaders and help you work with internal and cross-sector teams and organizations as well as communities who are hungry for change in their systems. It will provide the support necessary to bolster collaborative efforts focused on upstream determinants and long-term impacts and adapted or new systems that drive health and equity and are built co-creatively with partners and users.

Understanding Systems Change and How to Lead It

Key concepts we draw from and explore in this book include systems change and leading systems change. As described earlier, we use "systems change" to mean not just change in human behavior but change in the underlying structures and assumptions that drive it. This perspective on social change was developed by Donella Meadows as the Iceberg Model and was described in her posthumous book[5] and then adapted by Peter Senge.[6] At "the tip of the iceberg" are the events we observe. Below the "water" and not as evident are the underlying patterns of behavior that shape those events; below that are the organizational and social structures that constrain those patterns of behavior (including the dynamic processes that systems dynamics analysts illustrate with causal loops and stocks and flows); and below that are mental models that are largely unconscious but shared by members of a culture or community. The deeper we travel from the top of the iceberg, the more difficult it may be to effect change. Change at those lower levels of organizational and social structure and mental models, however, can result in radical and long-lasting change in patterns of behavior and the ways events unfold.

Taking this view of systems change means that "leading" systems change is something different than a command-and-control model of directing events or telling people to change their behavior—which frequently is not successful. No single individual can control social structures or mental models, so what do we mean by leading systems change? It requires a different mode of leadership and suggested steps that we set out in these pages. These include collective discussion and diagnosis of conditions at the lowest levels of the "iceberg," investigation of relationships within the structures and mental models, identification of accessible levers and opportunities for change and the resources to deploy them, working collaboratively with partners to utilize those levers, and building the personal leadership and relationships necessary for effective collaborative work.

Key Principles for Working With Systems Change

Guiding principles for systems change are woven throughout these chapters. They serve as touchstones that have shaped the choice of sources and the topics each author addresses. Our approach to creating this book was to bring together insights and practical tools that public health practitioners can use to further the work of leading systems change. Adapt and mold these principles to meet your needs—they lay a strong foundation on which to build your capacity for systems change leadership.

Health equity and racial and social justice is a key principle. We must utilize an equity lens in all our work, and this requires us to build this capacity in our workforce, in our relationships, on our teams, in our organizations, and in our work with communities. A second key principle is *personal leadership development*, including development of emotional intelligence as well as other personal leadership competencies such as a professional vision statement. A third key principle is *interpersonal leadership development*, including authentic engagement that treats others as whole and whole-hearted people. *Team leadership development*, including development of high-performing internal and external teams with strong communication skills, is a fourth key principle. *Community engagement*, including authentic engagement and co-creation with community members and other community stakeholders, is a fifth key principle. *Openness and learning* (not in the sense of being uncritical but of being open to learning), starting with "not knowing" or "beginner's mind" when listening to or observing others and the world, is a sixth key principle. This approach supports being aware of and learning about mental models and using discovery of differences and surprises in others' mental models to become more aware of your own. Through this openness and learning principle, you will begin to embrace the process of systems change leadership that includes examination of the root causes of the complex problems we face, development and implementation of solutions that include systems and structural change, and the sustainability of our change efforts. By practicing these six principles and using the tools provided, you will fine-tune your understanding and implementation or adaptation of the principles. You will find your approach to systems change leadership—as an individual, as a team, as an organization, and as a part of encompassing communities.

Defining Systems Thinking

There are many different traditions and schools of systems thinking. Some come from the desire to have a "theory of everything," from atoms to galaxies. Others are more relevant to practitioners who aim to lead desired change on human scales. We draw in this book from some recent and some not-so-recent models of systems thinking and leading change that we find clear and useful for public health practitioners. Kurt Lewin's work, though he wrote in the 1940s, continues to be practical, with his three-step model of change in organizations: unfreezing, change, (re-)freezing.[7] Linsky and Heifetz's *The Power of Adaptive Leadership* is seminal in making the distinction between technical leadership, limited by specific expert content knowledge, and adaptive leadership, which can handle complex human relationships and changing contexts.[8] More recently, Senge, Hamilton, and Kania described "The Dawn of System Leadership," affirming the importance of "the ability to see the larger system, fostering reflection and more generative conversations, and shifting the collective focus from reactive problem solving to cocreating the future."[4] What this means for public health practitioners is what we lay out in this book.

WHO IS THE AUDIENCE FOR THIS BOOK?

As mentioned earlier, this book is written for busy public health practitioners working in governmental public health, not-for-profit, and academia, as well as those who bring their public health expertise and passion to bear in the private sector. It is for those who work across industries, fields of study, and disciplines and have an interest in bringing a unique perspective to the table to help improve public health and well-being at the community or population level. It is for you if you live and work in a community and you care about improving the health of your community, even if you are not formally trained in public health. It is for those who want to dive deeper into the underlying issues that keep our long-standing public health challenges, such as racism, poverty, hunger, and homelessness, in place. It is for those who want to focus on the systems level challenges that make these very complex problems unyielding—and want to engage in systems level change in collaboration and coordination with others who care as deeply as you do.

Whether or not you currently are in a formal leadership role, this book is for you. Much like Heifetz and Linsky, authors of *The Power of Adaptive Leadership*,[8] we believe leadership is so much more than a role or title; it is a process, and it is our responsibility to bring our best selves, thinking, and actions to this process to make significant and necessary headway on complex public health challenges.

It is not uncommon for mid-career and senior-career professionals to find their way to systems change leadership work. If this is you, perhaps you can relate to conducting needs assessment after needs assessment, followed by one new program after another and evaluation after evaluation without evidence that you have transformed the public health outcomes that concern you. You know from experience that we need a new approach to solving our public health challenges. These chapters give you that approach. They provide strategies and tools that allow you to apply your public health expertise through a different lens—a systems change leadership lens.

If you are a student or new and emerging leader building your public health expertise—whether that be subject-matter expertise, such as maternal and child health, or technical expertise, such as needs assessment, program development, epidemiology, or data analysis—this book is worth your time and consideration. We need our new leaders to be subject-matter and technical experts in public health as well as individuals who can facilitate complex discussions with diverse stakeholders and work with them to align around common visions and agendas, goals, and action plans. We need people with the relational leadership capacity to facilitate the inevitable messiness that can happen when diverse and passionate people come together, each with a vision and ideas about improving public health. This is the place where the whole can become greater than the sum of its parts. If you can help facilitate the complexity, then we have the chance to create a magically new and evolved world that values all people the same.

If you are a brave and passionate person who is willing to take on systems change for the sake of making our world better, this book is for you. We need your passion, bravery, boldness, and commitment to evolving the exciting and ever-changing field of public health.

HOW IS THIS BOOK ORGANIZED?

The book's 15 chapters are organized into four sections: Framing Systems Change; The Levels and Success Practices for Systems Change in Public Health; The Process to Lead Systems Change; and Practical Examples. The book also includes a Preface by respected systems change leaders and an Afterword that inspires us to think bigger about systems change leadership for the future of our field.

Section I: Framing Systems Change

Section I includes three chapters. Chapter 1 is this introduction; it sets the stage with descriptions of what we mean by systems change, who the audience is for this book, how the book is organized, and how to use this book. Note that for our purposes, we refer to systems thinking, systems change, and leading systems change to mean the process by which we achieve systems change leadership. It is the process we use to thoroughly examine with diverse partners the root challenges of seemingly intractable public health problems and address them at a systems level. Chapter 2 shows you how to place racial justice and power-sharing at the heart of any systems change leadership work in which you engage. Here you will learn about how power imbalances, racism, and other forms of oppression define and structure the systems that drive health, how to "be" together versus "do" together to establish the deeper relationships needed to disrupt these systems, and how to embody power-sharing for systems transformation. Chapter 3 examines how to know if you are ready for systems change work. It also prefaces Section II with an overview of the different levels of systems change work on which to focus to ensure the best possible community-based work and community and population outcomes.

Section II: The Levels and Success Practices for Systems Change in Public Health

Section II includes Chapters 4 through 7. Chapter 4 discusses developing yourself as a leader, who you are as a leader, what you stand for, what difference you want to make in your work, and how to align with and lead with others. Here you will learn to develop emotional intelligence through articulating your vision and values as a leader. Chapter 5 presents a process to develop meaningful interpersonal relationships and strong interpersonal leadership. Here you will learn to engage with others and align your vision into a shared vision. You also will learn how best to communicate with colleagues and partners to build strong relationships. Chapter 6 looks at the changes we need to make in our organizational systems and structures to elevate the voices of those who often are silenced. This work includes applying a racial equity, access, diversity, and inclusion lens to modernizing our organizations. Chapter 7 focuses on development and facilitation of leadership to secure high-functioning teams. It highlights skills such as crucial conversations, conflict resolution, getting work done, action learning, and leading up and across. At the completion of Section II, you will have the understanding, plus tools and exercises, to build a strong foundation for systems change leadership in your organization and with your diverse stakeholders.

Section III: The Process to Lead Systems Change

Section III includes four chapters (Chapters 8 through 11). Chapter 8 addresses the important role of community partnership in leading systems change. The chapter highlights community organizing, coalition building, and engaging nontraditional partners in our public health work. Such nontraditional partners may include business, education, housing, transportation, or other sectors. Chapter 9 describes the process for identifying the root challenges associated with our complex public health challenges. This critical chapter implores us to take time to truly understand a problem before applying a (potentially unsuccessful) solution. Chapter 10 considers issues related to planning for systems change, managing the implementation of your change, and building in a process to learn and adapt as you go. Chapter 11 discusses practical sustainability concepts for your systems change leadership toolbox, including common facilitators and barriers to sustainability. At the completion of Section III, you will be able to actively engage in a systems change process, perhaps addressing a common problem by using a more holistic approach. This process likely will lead to different and more innovative solutions and new partnerships and resources.

Section IV: Practical Examples

Section IV includes Chapters 12 through 15. Chapter 12 sets the stage for highlighting a range of systems change leadership efforts presented in this section. This chapter features a community systems change effort with Feed the Children in New Orleans and a national systems change leadership effort with the National Consortium for Public Health Workforce Development. Chapter 13 provides systems change leadership examples at the state level in Florida focused on the state's Office of Children's Medical Services (CMS) Managed Care Plan and Specialty Programs and its Title V Children with Special Health Care Needs (CSHCN) Program, as well as four systems change leadership efforts at the local level, including examples from Oklahoma's OKC-County Health Department, the DuPage Health Department in Illinois, the Las Animas-Huerfano Counties Health Department in Colorado, and Minnesota's Saint Paul–Ramsey County Public Health. Chapter 14 presents a comprehensive systems change leadership example from Washington State that looks at K–12 school closings during COVID-19. Chapter 15 discusses applying a systems thinking approach to public health emergency and preparedness response, citing the example of efforts within

Cook County Department of Public Health in Illinois. Section IV provides a strong sense of the range of systems change leadership actions at national, state, local, and community levels. Hopefully, these examples will inspire your own thinking about systems change leadership, applying this approach to your own work.

What to Expect Across Chapters

We begin each chapter with an *introduction* that includes the learning objectives for the chapter. The *chapter objectives* provide the focus for each chapter and what you will learn by reading the chapter. Each chapter then provides the necessary *definitions* to ensure that we are speaking the same language around terms that may have multiple meanings. We present relevant, *evidence-based frameworks* to guide your thinking about the chapter content and provide the support you need to develop your work or secure buy-in to apply the content at work. We offer *public health practice-based examples* when possible to make chapter content more relevant to your work and to spark ideas about integrating the content into your organization. Each chapter offers *tools, exercises, practices, and/or steps* that you may apply to immediately begin to build experience with and ultimately expertise in systems change leadership work. We conclude each chapter with a *summary*—a synopsis of the chapter, key messages, tips, and supplemental resources that you may find useful as you undertake systems change leadership.

HOW TO USE THIS BOOK

While we recommend reading this book sequentially from front to back, we know that readers have great demands on their time. Each chapter is designed to stand alone and contains what you need to know within the chapter, including tools you can begin to engage with immediately. You do not need to read the previous chapter(s) to understand a selected chapter.

We encourage you to use the table of contents to find a section of the book or a chapter that speaks to you. Or flip to the end of a chapter to read a short summary. This will provide key messages from the chapter, immediately applicable tips, and supplemental resources that may directly address your needs or interests.

Try to practice right away with one or more of the recommended tools and reflect on your experience using the tool: What worked and what didn't? How might this tool support you to engage in your work differently and more systemically? How might this work support your team, your organization, and your community? There is no wrong or right way to work with tools. Work with them exactly as they are presented or adapt them to meet your needs; try them as soon as you can. We are committed to doing the work to develop ourselves as systems change leaders—don't let the suggested exercises sit in these pages, never to be practiced. Work with the content; learn from the content; grow with or adapt the content to meet your needs.

Reading this book with a group of colleagues in your organization is a good strategy for building a common language around systems change and systems thinking in support of improved systems change leadership. Consider reading the book with trusted colleagues from across organizations and sectors. Reflect on what systems change leadership means to you, your organization, your community, and public health. Engage with others to see how they view and experience systems change leadership similarly or differently than you do. Talk about systems change leadership. Reflect on how to take steps to be systems change leaders. Become the change you wish to see in the world.

REFLECTIONS FROM THE BOOK EDITORS

The content of this book and the process outlined for engaging in systems change leadership is based on systems science combined with our years of experience in leading systems change in our own public health practice work and in our academic work, including significant practice-based research in support of the education and development of public health practitioners all over the world. To complement our practical experience, we partnered with a range of highly respected chapter authors who have their own extensive practice-based expertise and experience with systems change leadership. Together, we provide you with our best thinking and experience about how to lead systems change in public health so that collectively we can develop systems that create the conditions for all people to be healthy.

While we have broad experience, our ability to fine-tune a shared language around systems change leadership is a work in progress. Our understanding of how to effectively do this work in practice is always and humbly being refined based on what we learn in collaboration with each new student, colleague, partner, and community member with whom we work.

As you read, the language around systems change leadership is evolving based on our collective, ongoing learning and in response to your needs and learnings from your own engagement in systems change leadership. Your active engagement in this work and sharing your process will shape the future of systems change leadership in public health and future iterations of these chapters. We hope you enjoy this book and find it valuable. Please share your comments and feedback with two of the book's editors: Christina Welter (cwelte2@uic.edu) and Kristina Risley (kris@krisrisley.com). If you sample the tools, practices, and exercises in these chapters, let us know about your successes and challenges. We look forward to hearing from you.

REFERENCES

1. Ison R. *Systems Practice: How to Act: In Situations of Uncertainty and Complexity in a Climate Change World.* 2nd ed. Springer Nature; 2017.
2. Williams B, Hummelbrunner R. *Systems Concepts in Action: A Practitioner's Toolkit.* Stanford University Press; 2011.
3. Midgley G. Systemic intervention for public health. *Am J Public Health.* 2006;96:466–472. doi:10.2105/AJPH.2005.067660.
4. Senge P, Hamilton H, Kania J. The dawn of system leadership. *Stanf Soc Innov Rev.* 2015;13(1):27–33. doi:10.48558/YTE7-XT62.

5. Meadows D. *Thinking in Systems: A Primer*. Chelsea Green Publishing; 2008.
6. Senge P. *The Fifth Discipline: The Art & Practice of the Learning Organization*. Doubleday, Random House; 2006.
7. Burnes B. The origins of Lewin's three-step model of change. *J Appl Behav Sci*. 2019;56(1): 32–59. doi:10.1177/0021886319892685.
8. Heifetz R, Grashow A, Linsky M. *The Practice of Adaptive Leadership: Tools and Tactics for Changing Your Organization and the World*. Cambridge Leadership Associates; 2009.

2

Racial Justice and Power-Sharing: The Heart of Leading Systems Change

Lili Farhang and Solange Gould

> "No one can define or measure justice, democracy, security, freedom, truth, or love. No one can define or measure any value. But if no one speaks up for them, if systems aren't designed to produce them, if we don't speak about them and point toward their presence or absence, they will cease to exist."
> —Donella Meadows[1(p177)]

CHAPTER OBJECTIVES

By the end of this chapter, practitioners will have learned the following core principles and capabilities to implement our approach, which are based on our experience working with over 100 health departments and public health organizations. These include:

- How to develop a shared analysis and expand our mental models regarding the manner in which power imbalances, racism, and other forms of oppression define and structure the systems that drive health.
- Attending to the work of "being" together, and not just "doing" together, as a way of deepening the relationships necessary to disrupt these patterns at the interpersonal, team, organizational, and community levels.
- Establishing change processes that embody a model of sharing power and shifting who represents and is leading transformation.

INTRODUCTION

Picture any social system: A school system. A food system. A tax system. A workplace. A healthcare setting. A city. An economy. Now, picture who has the power to decide how these systems operate. Picture who benefits from the system, who is harmed by or bears the brunt of its failures. When you really think about it, the picture shows that those with the power to decide are often quite distant from those who experience the system's harms and burdens. Power—the ability to enact change in the system—is not justly shared. People who bear the brunt of broken, inequitable systems—people receiving poorer healthcare, living in lower-quality housing, working in high-risk jobs, attending lower-resourced schools, and living with pollution and climate impacts, and those who are incarcerated— are the furthest from formal centers of power. And all these dynamics are racialized.

The people, families, and communities experiencing systemic harms and lacking access to power are primarily Black, Indigenous, Latinx, and other People of Color. And even when the system's harmful impacts and disempowerment are disproportion- ately felt by income, gender, sexuality, or other aspects of one's identity, the impacts are still racialized. All social systems have racially disparate outcomes.

Given that individual and community health status is determined by these living, working, and social conditions,[2] redressing disproportionate impacts and transform- ing these systems to be more equitable are central to achieving health equity. There is no question that the field of public health has this commitment[3] and has focused on improving the social determinants of health for several decades. Despite our best efforts, though, systems change to achieve health equity is often stymied by the same power imbalances and inequities that are present in the systems we seek to change; power structures resist change and hierarchies maintain privilege for some, at the ex- pense of others. Systems function to reproduce the power dynamics by which they are structured. And these dynamics show up at every level of our systems change efforts— interpersonal, team, organizational, and community.

Because of the fundamental ways that these entrenched dynamics endure and im- pede our progress toward health equity, this chapter comes early in this book. Leaders who are designing systems change processes must begin by accounting for these dy- namics at the outset—all other aspects of systems change leadership should flow from this. Our task is to attend to and overcome these patterns in order to change the poli- cies; practices; relationships; resource flows; and deeply held assumptions, values, and norms that make up all systems, including the public health system.

In that spirit, this chapter describes how systems change leaders can place the val- ues of racial justice and power-sharing at the heart of our practice, thereby shifting our own system in the process and supporting social movements to achieve systems change.

Describing Our Values of Racial Justice and Power-Sharing

Before diving into the core principles and capabilities, we want to ground practitioners in our North Star of what it means to share power and achieve racial justice.

Racial justice, which we interchangeably use with racial equity, is about deliberately transforming our systems to proactively serve those who have been most harmed by structural racism. As an outcome, racial justice is achieved when one's racial or ethnic identity no longer systematically exposes them to risks *or* no longer grants them privileges with regard to socioeconomic and life outcomes. It is when the people who need resources the most are prioritized to receive those resources. As a process, racial justice occurs when those most impacted by historic and current structural inequities are leading or are meaningfully engaged in systems change efforts.

Key to achieving racial justice is overcoming structural racism—a system of advantage based on race[4] in which racism is baked into policies, processes, and culture, across institutions and society over time. It is the cumulative and compounded effects of an array of factors, including public policies, institutional practices, cultural representations, and other norms that work in various and reinforcing ways to perpetuate racial inequity.[5]

We focus on dismantling racism and White supremacy because for nearly every indicator of health and well-being, there are differences by race, with Black, Indigenous, and People of Color (BIPOC) consistently faring worse than Whites. This holds true even when you look within other demographic characteristics such as income or gender. We lead with racial justice because every system that enables access to opportunity, health, and belonging was designed to reproduce racial inequities and continues to do so in the post-Civil Rights Era ubiquitously and often invisibly. And we lead with racial justice because chronic experiences of racism directly cause health inequities through the body's elevated stress response and consequent overexposure to cortisol and other stress hormones, which disrupt and depress almost all the body's processes. Experiences of discrimination and racial trauma can have intergenerational impacts on a family's health.[6] Finally, we lead with racial justice because of the urgent need to reckon with the United States' founding history of colonialism, genocide, and racial slavery; its continuation through Jim Crow; and its modern-day manifestations and sequelae, from intergenerational and persistent health inequities to disproportionate policing, incarceration, and state violence against BIPOC communities.

Other systems of advantage or oppression are also important to address in systems change, as inequities persist along all dimensions of identity, including income, gender, sexuality, immigration status, and more. But centering racial justice in systems change also leads to shifts in all forms of marginalization and supremacy. Racial justice provides us with the culture change, tools, lessons, and strategies to also undo the harmful effects of capitalism, patriarchy, and other systems bound up in systemic racism that advantage some at the expense of others.

Power-sharing means widening—and shifting—the circle of people involved in systems change and in centering people who are most impacted by inequities. There are many frameworks to understand what "power" is and how it operates. Power manifests in how decisions are made, the people and networks involved in the decisions, how problems and solutions are framed, and what ideas are even considered in a process. It comes in the form of resources, access to decision-making, alliances and networks, and the dominant stories society chooses to tell about this nation and its people.

Many people think of power as the "power over" that is used to oppress and cause harm. It is true that power imbalances lead to one group's enormous capacity to shape laws and government, dictate meaning, and actively repress anything that threatens their hold on that power. But as Dr. Martin Luther King Jr. stated, "*Power properly understood is nothing but the ability to achieve purpose. It is the strength required to bring about social, political, and economic change.*"[7(p37)] Power is not inherently good or bad—rather, its value depends on its locus, purpose, and manifestation. Perceiving power as "bad" can limit our ability to recognize that we have a role to play in pivoting its use toward good purposes. Systems change leaders must help groups clearly identify and perceive all of the locations and mechanisms of power, so that we can collectively and proactively use it to advance health equity.

Systems change is inherently about leveraging and shifting power within a system to bring about any desired change. Taking this a step further, the act of power-sharing must be understood as an end in and of itself in systems change. Given the manifold ways in which power-hoarding has led to systematic oppression of communities of color, the process of power-sharing in systems change helps set a new paradigm within the system itself. Any intervention to address structural racism is necessarily an intervention that shifts power.

DEVELOPING A SHARED ANALYSIS OF HOW POWER, RACISM, AND OTHER FORMS OF OPPRESSION PATTERN OUR SYSTEMS TODAY

How we understand the world is driven by our own mental models—our identity, our experiences, and our social position in existing systems. Our country's roots in White supremacy and racism have defined and limited our mental models. Brain science on implicit bias confirms that all our mental models and perceptions are limited by unconscious racial bias.[8] Coming together with others to develop a shared analysis of how a system operates is a hedge against any single entrenched or unconscious mental model dominating our systems change efforts. Indeed, developing a shared analysis of a system is a crucial first step of leading systems change and a prerequisite to developing solutions that actually solve systemic problems.

One aspect of unpacking our mental models and developing this shared analysis is understanding the "why" and the origin story of various systems' inequitable functioning. Every upstream system that drives health—education, criminal legal, housing, economic, and others—has a story about power, racism, and/or some other form of exclusion playing a role in the system's creation, function, and operation. To illustrate this, let's walk through a few examples of how historically racialized policies in our employment and housing sectors continue to yield inequitable outcomes today. This is what we mean by collaboratively "developing a shared analysis" to shift our mental models.

The National Labor Relations Act and the Fair Labor Standards Act—both cornerstones of employment and safety protections for workers today—have their roots in the preservation of strict racist hierarchies. Passed in 1935, domestic and agricultural workers were explicitly left out of these federal labor and employment laws,[9] which guarantee the right of private sector employees to organize into unions, engage in collective bargaining, and take collective action such as strikes. While these laws protect the health of many American workers today, they continue to exclude many others. The exclusions were intentional, dating back to the New Deal Era when Franklin D. Roosevelt (FDR) made concessions to gain the votes of Southern lawmakers seeking to exclude majority Black domestic and agricultural workers from the landmark laws. The power these lawmakers exerted in the political system was inextricably linked to a racist ideology that devalued Black life, sought to enrich and empower Whites, and led to the creation and continuation of deep and entrenched inequities in occupational safety and health outcomes. These exclusions remain today, and the racialized impacts and health harms remain for the immigrant and Latinx populations who now make up the bulk of the domestic and agricultural workforce.

Similar patterns are evident in the Federal Housing Administration's (FHA) mortgage lending practices and policies dating to the 1930s. Celebrated for making homeownership accessible to White people by guaranteeing their loans, the FHA explicitly refused to back loans to Black people or those who lived near Black people.[10] These policies intentionally created wealth for White people while systematically excluding non-Whites from home ownership, with implications for accruing intergenerational wealth, accessing quality public schools, and producing urban disinvestment and segregation.

The dominant mental model regarding the New Deal is that FDR instituted labor, industrial, banking, housing, and other systems changes that helped end the Great Depression, reduced income inequality, and brought a generation into the middle class. But absent in this dominant story is how people of color, and specifically Black people, were systematically excluded from the benefits and intentionally harmed by these systems changes.

A creative and dynamic tool to help develop this kind of shared analysis is Lee Anne Bell's *Storytelling Project Model*[11]—the purpose of which is to help communities "discover, develop, and analyze stories about racism that can catalyze consciousness and commitment to action."[11(p8)] It describes four types of stories: (a) stock stories, (b) concealed stories, (c) resistance stories, and (d) emerging/transforming stories. According to Bell, the four story types are "connected and mutually reinforcing. Each story type leads into the next in a cycle that fills out and expands our understanding of and ability to creatively challenge racism. The story types provide language and a framework for making sense of race and racism through exploring the genealogy of racism and the social stories that generate and reproduce it."[11(pp17–18)] To learn more about the model and how to apply the tool, visit: https://organizingengagement.org/models/storytelling-project-model/.[11]

Explicitly establishing that racism is structural creates a necessary foundation for change. It pinpoints the national, state, and local histories that created the systems we seek to change and so points to specific solutions. It normalizes discussions and thoughts that some people might be thinking but are afraid to say aloud. It takes the onus off any single individual or community to raise the pain of these stories and their impacts. It creates a "container" or process to name our individual and community experiences and validates the telling of those stories.

The legacy of racism, exclusion, and hoarding of power and resources is painful and lives in a deeply personal way in all of us today. To develop a shared analysis of the problem and its consequences and identify leverage points, systems change leaders must guide us to examine this history—and ask how these same dynamics influence the system today. As public health practitioners constantly seeking to "move upstream," this process helps us dismantle the individual behavior change approach that has permeated and stymied our health discourse and practice for decades. It helps us shift our attention to the roots of the problem, see the whole system, and comprehend the scale of changes necessary to remedy inequities.

CHANGING HOW WE "BE" TOGETHER TO TRANSFORM WHAT WE "DO" TOGETHER

> *"Real change starts with recognizing that we are part of the systems we seek to change. The fear and distrust we seek to remedy also exist within us—as do the anger, sorrow, doubt, and frustration."*
> —Peter Senge, Hal Hamilton, and John Kania[12(p29)]

The same power dynamics and hierarchies that arrange value based on race, gender, class, and other dimensions of identity are present in the systems we want to change *and* in the interpersonal, team, organizational, and community relationships that drive systems change. Leaders of systems change are thus charged with transforming a seemingly "external" system, while also transforming the sociocultural dynamics—including ways of being in our teams—that we all have internalized and that block real transformation.

This may cause alarm for some public health practitioners: *If we aren't about individual behavior change anymore, why are we focusing on changing people?* The answer is that systems leaders must foster collective leadership and ownership of the system and build the capacity of individuals, teams, and organizations to change the system. People created and maintain these systems, and it will take transformed people and relations to shift the systems. We need to shift people's perspectives and relationships within the system because expanded perspectives and relationships allow us to enact systems change more profoundly and effectively, and ultimately make transformation stick.

The heart of this work, therefore, is to design change processes that *in and of themselves* challenge status quo dynamics—to support a different way of "being together" that prioritizes relationship development, trust building, and bringing our whole selves to the work of changing the systems. For us, this comes down to two core practices: (a) creating a "container" for our work together and (b) reintegrating the head and the heart. In short, these ideas are what we mean when we put the values of racial justice and power-sharing into practice in our relationships. Let's dive into what this means.

Creating a "Container" for Our Work Together

Systems leaders must create the conditions that give rise to change and allow change to become self-sustaining. In practice, we call this "creating a container for systems change processes." Creating a container is about constructing a shared working and thinking space that allows for an equitable set of dynamics and culture to emerge to help us tackle complex problems. This container acknowledges that we are all harmed by unjust systems and prepares us to be simultaneously vulnerable, afraid, and brave.

In practice, the container is about:

- establishing collective practices for people to share their personal stories, identities, and vulnerabilities;
- creating group agreements to guide how people communicate with one another, especially on charged topics;
- explicitly naming and holding the physical and emotional dysregulation that invariably comes with doing racial justice and systems change work;
- giving room for a group to slow down and notice when they are having an emotional or body response to the content; and
- creating a "physical" space that grounds relationships, which includes accessible room set-up, welcoming music, what's on the walls, shared food, and prioritizing time for wellness and joy.

To learn more about these practices, check out Human Impact Partners' "Container Setting" tool in our health equity tools and resources: https://humanimpact.org/products-resources/.[13]

Attention to the container helps create an environment that humanizes the process and participants and builds greater social and emotional intelligence. It helps build trust among a group undertaking systems change, which is the foundation for greater innovation—and critical for overcoming public health's risk aversion. As this is fundamentally counter to the "professional" culture into which many of us have been trained, it is also an interruption of the systemic status quo unto itself. Importantly, it is about creating a space for accountability for feedback mechanisms that are available to everyone, irrespective of the power they hold within the change process. A well-curated and held container creates processes and spaces where people feel they belong and where there is a shared set of rules and capacity to work through the interpersonal, team, and organizational conflict that is inherent in systems change.

Reintegrating the Head and the Heart

Our commitment to racial justice also requires a capacity and willingness to feel the work we are doing—in an embodied sense, in addition to the intellectual. "Integrating the head and the heart" is a metaphor for making space in our work for the physical sensations and emotions that arise when we confront the reality of racial inequities and unjust power imbalances, both in the policies and systems we want to shift and in our own organizational culture.

Public health has been acculturated to approach health equity work with a primary focus on policy change, planning, analyzing, and producing data—and other activities primarily "of the head." In the United States, nearly all of us carry trauma in our bodies from racism and White supremacy. We have tended to suppress the visceral pain and trauma of living through, witnessing, and perpetuating systems of oppression and advantage. We must break down this false dichotomy between thinking and feeling. In practice, this means:

- developing an ever-evolving vocabulary and collective analysis about what it means to be heart-centered,
- normalizing the practice of noticing and being able to share whether we are emotionally regulated or not as we engage with this work,
- making space for shared reflection about how a body of work affects us as people,
- listening deeply to those who have been most impacted,
- considering how we ourselves have suffered the trauma of participating and living within harmful systems, and
- breathing together more, paying attention to how our bodies feel, and developing a vocabulary to express what's happening there as we engage in this work.

To learn how to bring these practices into change processes, check out adrienne maree brown's visionary book, *Emergent Strategy: Shaping Change, Changing Worlds*,[14] at: www.akpress.org/emergentstrategy.html. It is an excellent resource on inviting people engaged in systems change to "feel, map, assess, and learn from the swirling patterns around us in order to better understand and influence them as they happen."[15] Similarly, Brené Brown's seminal work on vulnerability, putting yourself out there, and courage are excellent resources—visit her extensive library of videos, tools, and resources here: https://brenebrown.com/.[16] The daring leading assessment tool and the workbook for groups to operationalize their values are particularly useful.

Systems change leaders understandably face significant pressures to succeed from stakeholders, all of whom leverage some form of power. The pressure to "act" or "do" is ever present, as people's lives and well-being depend on transforming the conditions that cause harm. Leaders who are engaged in transformational work may believe resources are being "wasted" to dedicate valuable staff time to "internal work" that does not directly address community needs. But the dichotomy between internal practices and external work is a false one. We cannot achieve equitable outcomes without recognizing that power dynamics and structural racism rest on the formalization of often-undissected implicit interpersonal codes, workplace hierarchies, and professional practices that mirror and perpetuate inequities. Indeed, genuine systems change must begin within. Ultimately, we need to feel that trauma in order to bring our whole selves to systems change work with humility, vulnerability, and honesty.

Even in organizations working explicitly on racial justice and health equity, we have seen how harmful internal culture and practices can foment distrust between staff, leadership, organizations, and communities; derail plans; and waste substantial resources and time. This leads to further demoralization, cynicism, loss of trust, and difficulty recruiting and retaining BIPOC staff and racial equity champions. A work culture that fosters ongoing reflection and collaboration and prioritizes the well-being of all participants and relationships is central to sustaining systems change efforts—not an optional "nice to have" or one-off. During this unprecedented year of a global pandemic, police murders and brutality, climate change impacts, and the rise of White supremacist extremist groups and militants, we have directly witnessed how investing in how we "be together" at work profoundly impacts our ability to weather the chaos, show up for each other, pivot in changing conditions, support social movements and power building, and continue to facilitate policy and systems change. When we establish new patterns of being together in our systems change efforts, we are better equipped to do "the work."

MODELING POWER-SHARING AND CENTERING THOSE MOST IMPACTED WITHIN THE SYSTEMS CHANGE PROCESS

Leading systems change thinker Donella Meadows instructs us to identify "leverage points" as the points of power in a given system.[17] Leverage points include the power to set the rules of the system, to change or evolve the structure of the system, to set the goals and paradigm of the system, and—most critically—to *transcend* the paradigm of the system.

Communities facing health and social inequities—for example, students in underperforming schools, families living in poor quality housing, workers subsisting on poverty wages, communities that are policed and incarcerated—rarely have access to these leverage points *by design*. Community engagement opportunities should define these leverage points and redistribute the power toward those who have been most disenfranchised.[18]

Power-Sharing in the Systems Change Process Itself

In systems change processes, leaders have enormous ability to influence how power and leverage are exercised—for example, how we perceive the problem; how goals, rules, structure, and recourse are decided and by whom; the given options for systems change solutions; and how the paradigm or system will ultimately shift. Systems change efforts are relational and involve negotiations between actors and agents of change with varying degrees of power—supervisors and supervisees, public agencies and people who rely on public services, corporations and workers. Transforming systems requires transforming the balance of power and relationships among people who shape and experience the systems. One tool to do this is "power analysis" or "power mapping," which helps those seeking social change to analyze who holds power over decision-making, the influence they have, and how to target them for change. To learn more about power analysis/mapping and see an example, visit: https://commonslibrary.org/guide-power-mapping-and-analysis/.[19]

A power-sharing approach to systems change requires systems actors to meaningfully shift their dominant role or position in the system, with some actors relinquishing control or authority and those with less leverage stepping into greater ownership and responsibility. A power-sharing approach reflects a more mutual and interdependent model for pulling on the levers of change, as opposed to sticking with an old paradigm of those with existing power continuing to dominate.

Ultimately, power-sharing means widening and shifting who is involved in sense-making, setting the rules of the system, and determining the set of options from which to choose (i.e., the paradigm of the system). Focusing on shifting power in systems change is necessary to ensure that other aspects of systems change—that is, changing policies, practices, resource flows, and norms—will ultimately be retained.

Changing Who Is at the Table to Center Those Who Are Most Impacted

Power-sharing in systems change is inextricably tied to racial justice via who is represented in change processes. Changing who is at the systems change table—and transforming that table—is itself a strategy to remedy the historic and ongoing injustices that have intentionally excluded BIPOC from decision-making. In addition to this reparative effect, changing who is at the table has a substantive impact on the conversations we have, the choices we consider, and the transformation we pursue. It is about much more than representation—it is about bringing deep expertise, specificity, and definition of root causes and impacts to the systems change process.

Community power-building organizations (i.e., grassroots community organizations) that are made up of and represent people and communities most impacted by inequities are a natural ally for systems leaders seeking to change who is at the table, address racial inequities, and integrate a power-sharing model. Community power-building organizations focus on redistributing power and decision-making by building power in communities most impacted by economic, political, social, health, and other inequities. They use diverse tactics and movement strategies to engage communities, bring them together to build a shared analysis across their lived experiences and conditions, and take collective action. They understand the process of building power at a local scale, within historically marginalized communities, as having the potential to transform how decisions are made—by, with, and for whom—on a larger scale. See the article "Shifting and Sharing Power: Public Health's Charge in Building Community Power" in *NACCHO Exchange* for seven concrete tips on how health departments can work with community power-building organizations: www.humanimpact .org/shiftsharepower.[20]

What would it mean to bring formerly incarcerated people and abolitionists into discussions about policing and incarceration, or renters and unhoused people into discussions about housing affordability, or people experiencing wage theft into discussions about regulating workplaces? The expertise and specific information of their navigation of systems and experiences will lead the way to transformative solutions. These may not be easy solutions to implement—but then, if they were, they wouldn't be transformative.

A NEW PARADIGM TO STRUCTURE OUR SYSTEMS

In this chapter, we've described what it means to place racial justice and power-sharing at the heart of systems change. In practice, this is about creating a shared analysis of how racism, power imbalances, and other forms of oppression structure our systems today; about changing how we are in relationship with one another and with ourselves; and about modeling power-sharing and centering the voices of people who have been most impacted by the systems we seek to change. This topic has many more aspects than we were able to cover in one chapter, but we believe these are the core capabilities central to leading effective and transformative systems change at the interpersonal, team, organizational, and community levels.

We are in the midst of a racial reckoning in this country, and too many people have been killed, injured, and harmed by unjust systems. Yet, because of the powerful racial justice movement work of BIPOC communities, we are also seeing unprecedented support for the movement for Black liberation, along with long-overdue introspection by many White people about their complicity in unjust systems and the necessity to be proactively antiracist. Because racism so deeply structures all systems, we *cannot* transform systems without this reckoning. And we need a vast network of brave systems change leaders and movers to guide us toward truth and reconciliation, justice, health, and abundance.

This is a process with no end, and no set arrival point. It is a constant state of change that adapts to new information and that gains wisdom and insight from dynamic conditions and perspectives. It acknowledges the status quo and opposing racist forces working to block equity-driven systems change. Conflict is inherent to this process of transformation and should be welcomed as a sign of change and growth. Shifting power to be collectively dispersed across people and communities and toppling the hierarchies that assign value based on identity or social positionality is no easy process. But our mutual liberation and transformation depends on it.

CHAPTER SUMMARY

This chapter walks through how systems change leaders can place the values of power-sharing and racial justice at the heart of our systems change practices. Readers will understand the importance of a key set of core principles and capabilities central to leading effective and transformative systems change at the interpersonal, team, organizational, and community levels.

Key Messages

1. It is critical to expand our mental models and develop a shared analysis about how power imbalances, racism, and other forms of oppression define and pattern the systems that drive health.

2. We must attend to the work of "being" together and not just "doing" together as an important way of deepening the relationships necessary to disrupt these patterns at the interpersonal, team, organizational, and community levels.
3. We must establish change processes that are themselves a model of sharing power and shifting who represents and is leading transformation of our systems.

Tips

In order to operationalize these principles and capabilities, we offer these practical tips:

- Facilitate processes for groups engaged in systems change processes to examine the histories of racism, power imbalances, supremacy, and harm—and ask how these same dynamics influence the system today—to develop a shared analysis of the problem and its consequences and to identify leverage points.
- Create a container for systems change processes—a shared working and thinking space that allows for a different set of relational dynamics and culture to emerge, which can help tackle complex problems.
- "Integrate the head and the heart" to make space alongside our intellectual work to feel the physical sensations and emotions that arise when confronting the reality of racial inequities and unjust power imbalances—both in the policies and systems we aim to shift and in our own organizational culture.
- Adopt a power-sharing approach, where systems actors shift their dominant role, positionality, or component of the system, often relinquishing control and authority. This means taking a more mutual and interdependent approach and opening up opportunities for those with less leverage and power to step into greater ownership and responsibility.
- Change who is at the table to directly address racial inequities and integrate a power-sharing model by forging long-term relationships with community power-building organizations that often represent and are made up of people and communities most impacted by inequities.

Supplemental Resources

- Lee Ann Bell. *Storytelling for Social Justice: Connecting Narrative and the Arts in Antiracist Teaching.* Available at: www.routledge.com/Storytelling -for-Social-Justice-Connecting-Narrative-and-the-Arts-in-Antiracist/Bell/p/ book/9781138292802
- adrienne maree brown. *Emergent Strategy: Shaping Change, Changing Worlds.* Available at: www.akpress.org/emergentstrategy.html
- Brené Brown, LLC. *Dare to Lead Hub.* Available at: brenebrown.com/
- Cyndi Suarez. *The Power Manual: How to Master Complex Power Dynamics.* Available at: www.cyndisuarez.com/
- Grassroots Policy Project. *The Three Faces of Power.* Available at: www .grassrootspolicy.org/wp-content/uploads/2018/05/GPP_34FacesOfPower.pdf

- Human Impact Partners. *Heart-Centered Practice: Embodying a Racial Justice Framework.* Available at: www.humanimpact-hip.medium.com/heart-centered-practice-embodying-a-racial-justice-framework-1e8b32d0e7d
- Human Impact Partners. *Shifting and Sharing Power: Public Health's Charge in Building Community Power.* NACCHO Exchange. Available at: www.humanimpact.org/shiftsharepower
- Human Impact Partners. *Health Equity Tools.* Available at: www.humanimpact.org/products-resources/issue-area/?filter=iss1-145
- Racial Equity Institute. *The Groundwater Approach: Building a Practical Understanding of Structural Racism.* Available at: www.racialequityinstitute.com/groundwaterapproach
- Smithsonian Magazine. *158 Resources to Understand Racism in America.* Available at: www.smithsonianmag.com/history/158-resources-understanding-systemic-racism-america-180975029/

REFERENCES

1. Meadows D. *Thinking in Systems: A Primer.* Chelsea Green Publishing; 2008.
2. *County Health Rankings Model.* Robert Wood Johnson Foundation and the University of Wisconsin Population Health Institute. https://www.countyhealthrankings.org/explore-health-rankings/measures-data-sources/county-health-rankings-model. Accessed February 9, 2021.
3. *10 Essential Public Health Services.* de Beaumont Foundation and Public Health National Center for Innovations. https://spark.adobe.com/page/Qy1veOhGWyeu5/. Accessed February 9, 2021.
4. Wellman DT. *Portraits of White Racism.* 2nd ed. Cambridge University Press; 1993.
5. *Living Glossary for Racial Justice, Equity & Inclusion.* Southern Jamaica Plain Health Center and Racial Reconciliation and Healing. https://docs.google.com/document/d/1acNIuGSKAJLWYwzCa0TtKciftWE8iKb4vJZdcGW4zqw/edit. Accessed December 21, 2020.
6. Williams DR, Lawrence JA, Davis BA. Racism and health: Evidence and needed research. *Annu Rev Public Health.* 2019;40(1):105–112. doi:10.1146/annurev-publhealth-040218-043750.
7. King Jr, ML. *Where Do We Go From Here: Chaos or Community?* Beacon Press; 1968.
8. *Project Implicit.* https://implicit.harvard.edu/implicit/. Accessed January 13, 2021.
9. Katznelson I. *When Affirmative Action Was White.* W.W. Norton & Company; 2006.
10. Rothstein R. *The Color of Law: A Forgotten History of How Our Government Segregated America.* Liveright Publishing Corporation; 2017.
11. Bell LA. *Storytelling for Social Justice Connecting Narrative and the Arts in Antiracist Teaching.* 2nd ed. Routledge; 2020.
12. Senge P, Hamilton H, Kania J. The dawn of system leadership. *Stanf Soc Innov Rev.* 2015;13(1):27–33. doi:10.48558/YTE7-XT62.
13. *Capacity Building "Container Building" Approach + Practices.* Human Impact Partners. https://humanimpact.org/products-resources/. Accessed February 19, 2021.
14. brown am. *Emergent Strategy: Shaping Change, Changing Worlds.* AK Press; 2017.

15. brown am. *Emergent Strategy: Shaping Change, Changing Worlds.* https://www.akpress.org/emergentstrategy.html

16. Brené Brown, LLC. *Dare to Lead Hub.* https://brenebrown.com/. Accessed February 19, 2021.

17. Meadows D. *Leverage Points: Places to Intervene in a System.* The Sustainability Institute; 1998.

18. Arnstein SR. A ladder of citizen participation. *J Am Plann Assoc.* 1969;35(4):216–224. doi:10.1080/01944366908977225.

19. Tang A. *Power Mapping and Analysis.* The Commons Social Change Library. https://commonslibrary.org/guide-power-mapping-and-analysis/. Accessed February 19, 2021.

20. Farhang L, Gaydos M. *Shifting and Sharing Power: Public Health's Charge in Building Community Power.* NACCHO Exchange. http://www.humanimpact.org/shiftsharepower. Accessed February 19, 2021.

3

Facilitating Readiness for Systems Change

Amy Mullenix, Rebecca Wells, and Karen Trierweiler

CHAPTER OBJECTIVES

By the end of this chapter, the practitioner will be able to:

- Define change readiness.
- Understand the connection between learning organizations and change readiness.
- Understand how change conversations and more formal readiness assessments can be used to both measure and build readiness for change.
- Describe several aspects of readiness that intersect with change implementation, such as resistance.

INTRODUCTION

Public health change leadership is both challenging and crucial. Leaders in the field shoulder high levels of societal responsibility and often feel a moral imperative to protect the health of entire populations. They commonly work in the contexts of narrow decision-making authority, limited community understanding of public health, and constrained resources. Leadership must balance this context with the constant need to be ready for change.

In this chapter we explore change readiness concepts and several tools to consider for this purpose, many of which you may already use in your daily work. The ideas in this chapter can help you consider your organization's readiness to undertake and implement change at the individual, organizational, and systems levels. We describe the advantage of learning organizations in being ready for change, readiness tools such as change conversations and more formal readiness assessments, and finally offer some thoughts on leadership for readiness and resistance to change. A synthesis of how these concepts are connected to one another can be found at the end of the chapter in Figure 3.1.

DEFINING CHANGE READINESS

Readiness for change and the resulting change itself is the essence of Lewin's[1] "transition state," the space between the current state and a desired future state. In preparing to move forward from the current state, three intersecting and dynamic components of change readiness have been identified by Scaccia et al.,[2] which together describe a simple model that allows leaders to plan for and implement change. These three elements are represented as $R=MC^2$, where **R**eadiness = **M**otivation x general organizational **C**apacity and specific **C**apacity to undertake the change under consideration. These three elements can be present or absent in varying degrees within your organization and will vary depending on the culture of the organization, the complexity of the change at hand, the degree to which the current state is "broken" or not, the length of time you and your team have been considering a change, and many other factors. When considering any systems change, it is important for you as a leader to pause and consider the motivation and capacity currently in place in your organization and whether additional work is needed to be ready for the change ahead.

This readiness formula reinforces the idea described elsewhere in this book that change is both dynamic and iterative, and readiness as a component of systems change is fluid and depends on the motivation and capacity of your organization.

CASE EXAMPLE

A hypothetical case example is provided in the following and is used throughout the chapter to illustrate how leaders might enhance readiness to both plan and implement change. To mirror common real-life scenarios, the case example includes goals and complex system contexts, such as braided funding, historically siloed work, and staff fears of loss of status or control, that are mostly beyond public health leaders' control. Such contexts necessitate clarifying how a given organization's goals relate to those of stakeholders in local or state government, service providers, advocacy organizations, and the populations served.[3]

Case Study

CASE EXAMPLE: COMPREHENSIVE FUNDING FOR HEALTH EQUITY

Maria directs the Prevention Division at a state health department. She is responsible for all statewide prevention programs, organized within the following bureaus: Maternal Child Health; Chronic Disease; Tobacco Control; and Injury Prevention and Substance Use Prevention, including opioids. Most of the Prevention Division's funding comes from federal sources specific to the content or disease. Division leaders also work with local public health departments and community-based organizations that partner to meet the goals and objectives of federal funding.

Maria and some of her colleagues would like to establish a comprehensive community-based funding initiative to address health equity. This would require aggregating all of the program-specific funds, usually allocated by each of the bureaus in the department to a county, public health district, or region. These combined funds would then allow a specific community to address a wide range of issues and health problems that contribute to health inequities.

Clarifying the Prevention Division's readiness for the more comprehensive approach, Maria envisions assessing how motivated other stakeholders are to make the necessary changes, what the Division's overall capacity for change implementation is, and what the Division's capacity is relative to this particular initiative. For instance, it is possible that there is a shared passion for more integrated approaches to equity, and the Division has a strong track record of implementing new programs, but it does not have the legal or information systems wherewithal to integrate funding from different external sources.

LEARNING AS READINESS

In organizations, as in individuals, learning is essential to change. This concept has been described by Peter Senge[2] and built upon by many others. And, as organizations are composed of people, understanding your own and others' motivations and capacities is foundational to increasing organizational readiness. Thus, you as a leader can develop a plan to create your own change skills as well as foster these skills in the people you supervise and support. In addition, you can develop and sustain systems to combine individual learning into team learning and new processes.

Building both individual and team readiness using the five hallmarks of a learning organization[2] described in the following facilitates change planning and implementation when new opportunities and threats arise. Organizations and systems that display some or all of the five hallmarks of a learning organization have a readiness advantage in that learning organizations are essentially in a constant state of self-assessment. However, if your organization does not currently support all (or even some) of these hallmarks, this does not mean that change will be impossible, but instead that more readiness work will be required prior to the change.

1. **Personal mastery**
   Personal mastery of learning-related skills is a key component of organizational learning. This includes learning new things, trying new approaches, and "failing forward." Such individual growth becomes more possible when you as a leader model a learning orientation, support staff training and education, and actively value the new skills and ideas such opportunities generate. In turn, your organization can then become more ready for change as the team members develop experience applying new processes.
2. **Team learning**
   Team learning values learners and learning in all parts of the system. Collaboration is critical as platforms and infrastructure are built to support and share learning across your organization and even broader systems. This may involve your support for online learning repositories or structures such as regular meetings, convened with the purpose of discussing how both previous experiences and new insights might inform proposed change efforts. In cross-sector change efforts, a key role of leaders is to provide sufficient time for cross-sector learning, which might include activities such as intentionally building shared vocabularies and establishing norms across various organizations and/or sectors of a change initiative.
3. **Shared vision**
   Systems and organizations that drive successful change efforts are often supported by leaders who effectively communicate a shared vision for change. These leaders actively support innovation and build structures in which partners can participate authentically. This environment and a shared vision can produce motivation, which in turn builds readiness for change.
4. **Systems thinking**
   Systems thinking is a practice used to explore and document how things are connected to each other within some notion of a whole entity.[4] In a learning organization, your role as a leader can be to support individuals to actively connect their own work to broader societal trends and to initiatives that either align or contrast with your organization's goals. Systems thinking skills are particularly useful in building readiness for a particular change initiative, as you can be specific about how the potential change is connected to a broader whole.

   In public health, systems thinking can be particularly helpful in advancing health equity and other non traditional determinants of health. For instance, in the case example, using systems thinking to build readiness within the organization could lead to intentional choices about which community entities are best positioned to move equity efforts forward and, thus, are most worthy of funding. In addition, fostering systems thinking across departmental silos can result in organically derived plans for addressing equity more holistically across strict programmatic lines.
5. **Clear mental models**
   Mental models (our individual cognitive representations of the world around us) underlie all change efforts, and in cross-sector systems change efforts, one

role of leaders is to make sure that these individual models, or assumptions, are brought to the surface. Otherwise change might proceed with unspoken assumptions and quickly run into friction. Leaders can use specific tools such as causal loop diagrams to explicitly articulate and clarify mental models, resulting in clearer understanding of the problem at hand and increased readiness for change.

Learning organizations actively use some or all of these five hallmarks, and as a result are essentially building readiness for change on an ongoing basis. The notions of innovation and quality improvement come to function as cultural norms, and these organizations have the capacity in place to respond to proposed changes. For example, if a learning organization will be implementing the case example, those involved may view the proposed restructuring of funding mechanisms more favorably, given a track record of success in their organization's past learning and innovation efforts. Although all are not necessary for effective change, each of these learning hallmarks supports either motivation or capacity, which in turn supports organizational or individual readiness for change and promotes successful implementation.

Regardless of where your organization is in the learning process, the readiness assessment tools discussed in this chapter can help you and your partners prepare to facilitate readiness for systems change.

USING CHANGE CONVERSATIONS FOR READINESS

Your active leadership can support preparation for systems change at all levels of the organization, keeping in mind that efforts are most likely to be successful when participants have time to prepare at the individual, team, and organizational levels. Change conversations can be used as an informal readiness assessment. They are based on reflective questioning and can be used to enhance motivation and capacity for change.[5] They might most effectively be used at the team or organizational level, so that individuals have the benefit of listening to and learning from the perspective of others. In systems change efforts, you can think of these conversations as on the spectrum of readiness assessments somewhere between learning organizations' innate readiness capacity and formal readiness assessment tools described later in the chapter.

Change Conversations:
Who—What—When—Where—Why—How

The "why and when" conversations begin to articulate the idea that some aspect of the current situation may not be advancing the organizational vision/mission or, in the case of a broader systems change, the goals of a broader initiative. This conversation can often be bolstered with data that demonstrate your current approach is not getting to the outcomes you desire, and you can use question prompts such as:

- Are our current activities achieving the outcomes we desire?
- Might we want to lead or participate in broader systems-level or upstream efforts to help us attain the desired outcomes?
- When would this happen?
- Are we ready?
- What would we need to do to get ready?

These conversations can provide intellectual and motivational rationales for a different path forward (i.e., the future state). If used strategically with other change conversations, articulating the "why and when" for systems change can increase motivation and result in individual and organizational buy-in for systems change.

The "why" conversation is particularly critical in building "buy-in" for the change described in the case example. Public health has long embraced the concept of health equity as vitally important, yet concrete efforts to demonstrate significant changes in outcomes have been lacking. The importance of acting on this critical public health issue serves as a compelling "why" in support of change.

Closely related to "why and when," the "where and what" refers to "where are we going and what might we do to get there" conversations—leader descriptions that paint an aspirational picture of the future state, highlighting the benefits to the target population (the system as a whole) and to individuals and teams as change leaders. If changes are expected at the systems level, beyond the organization, this connection to the broader systems structure is critical to convey to enhance readiness for change. Over time, change participants become motivated (and thereby more ready for change) as their depth of understanding increases about the ultimate goals and the organization's role in the systems change.

In "who" and "how" conversations, leaders describe the proposed change process, partnerships, and timeline. Here it is critical for you as a leader to be transparent about who is expected to contribute, and in what ways, to the change process, and whether the final decision-making processes will be collaborative or will consider input from all participants but ultimately rest with a few individuals. These conversations can also include your ideas about the organization's readiness that have already emerged from other readiness assessments and more informal ongoing organizational learning.

There is no one best way to approach these change conversations, but framing them as shared learning opportunities rather than using a top-down approach is more likely to garner momentum for the proposed change and enhance readiness. Your role as the leader in these conversations is to adopt and model a learning posture, while still being willing to push the team beyond the status quo. Over time these conversations can build trust in your leadership and motivation for systems change. As change conversations progress, everyone involved in the change should be able to answer these questions: What might this potential change mean for me in my role? What might the change mean for my team? My organization? The way our organization interacts with other players in the broader system?

USING SEMI-FORMAL READINESS ASSESSMENTS TO INCREASE MOTIVATION AND CAPACITY FOR SYSTEMS CHANGE

If not part of an advanced learning organization, semi-formal readiness assessments can help you as a leader to understand where the "pain points" of a given change effort are most likely to emerge. These assessments are used in planning for systems change and generally involve group activities in which team members reflect on their own motivation and capacity to undertake a systems-level change. In addition to learning about your team or organization's internal capacity for systems change, readiness assessments by their very nature can also be tools that prepare organizations or individuals to both plan for and implement change.

For example, as public health systems move away from programs that serve specific populations toward initiatives led by community organizations, public health goals are now shifting toward comprehensive community-level improvements rather than small-scale improvements for special populations or those targeted to a narrow set of outcomes. As illustrated in the case scenario, where practitioners in particular programs have been responsible for program implementation with a specific population for many years, a formal readiness assessment might alert leaders to the fact that these individuals may resist efforts to move away from their special populations of interest. Knowing this in advance of a wide-scale change effort can help leaders provide learning opportunities about the benefits of community-led initiatives, and the efforts that will be needed to truly impact health equity across a given community.

Readiness assessments might also bring to light the fact that hiring choices might need to shift to better develop staff capability to support a particular type of change. In the case example, readiness assessments of the Division as a whole as well as of specific bureaus may surface concerns about the program's willingness to be led by different collaborators and to change the nature of their work, in some cases from individual interventions to population health initiatives. Staff capacity and beliefs about working in new ways could also be raised.

READINESS ASSESSMENT TOOLS

There are many types of readiness assessment tools described in the formal leadership literature that have been used to measure motivation and capacity at multiple levels. The $R=MC^2$ described earlier is one such model that has been proposed for use in this way. It describes readiness as a combination of motivation, general organizational capacity, and specific capacity to undertake the change under consideration.[2]

At the level of individual assessment, one basic activity that can be helpful is to ensure all team members have tools and time to reflect on their own change style. There are simple assessments available. One of the most common simple assessments is the

Change Style Indicator® (CSI®), a leadership assessment designed to measure an individual's preferred style in approaching and addressing change. It provides respondents with insights on personal preferences for managing through change. It also provides context for how those around them might perceive and respond to their preferred style. This assessment results in placement along a continuum of change style preference, from conserver to pragmatist to originator. With results in hand, all team members can process anticipated changes with knowledge of their own style, while also understanding that the styles and preferences of their colleagues may be complementary or contradictory to their own.

At the team or organizational level, you can use the change conversations as described earlier to informally assess the readiness of your team members and organization to embark on a new systems change. One strategy to formalize your learning from change conversations is to document the takeaways, hesitations, and momentum that emerge. You can then synthesize your observations about the organization's readiness for systems change and describe it for your organization for further discussion. You can also use these reflections to identify areas for further individual or organizational motivation or capacity building.

A more formal readiness assessment tool may also be useful at the organizational level, in conjunction with or to further explore learning that arises from change conversations. Again, many tools exist, but as a leader you and your team are likely already familiar and comfortable with the SWOT (strengths, weaknesses, opportunities, threats)[6,7] tool, often used for strategic planning. With a subtle shift of purpose, the SWOT can also be used to strategically assess readiness by uncovering change "facilitators" and "barriers" in a methodical way. The tool helps to document both internal and external forces that are likely to push the change forward as well as resist it. As part of the SWOT process, many ideas are likely to emerge related to specific potential changes that would leverage the organization's strengths and/or compensate for organizational weaknesses.[7] In this sense, the readiness assessment also becomes a space for co-creation of change ideas within the organization.

When used for readiness assessment, the SWOT tool is highly flexible and familiar to most practitioners. It can be facilitated just one time with a leadership team as part of a regular meeting, or many times with multiple stakeholders in an organization. Exhibit 3.1 illustrates a readiness assessment SWOT, including guiding questions the session facilitator can ask to prompt discussion. It also includes the funding integration case example to illustrate how the SWOT analysis might be used to explore a specific potential change.

EXHIBIT 3.1 SWOT Tool for Readiness Assessment

Brief description of proposed change:

_____

Case example: State categorical funding will be re-purposed in alignment with federal and state rules and regulations to foster innovation and flexibility at the local level to directly reduce health inequities in a given community.

SWOT participants: _____

Date: _____

	CHANGE FACILITATORS	CHANGE IMPEDIMENTS
INTERNAL ASPECTS	**Strengths** • In what ways are we poised to make this change? *Case example*: Key state staff and local community organizations are supportive and ready to implement; there is general staff buy-in around the importance of health equity • What unique knowledge, talent, or resources do we have that might push this change forward? *Case example*: The Health Equity Learning Collaborative has been analyzing potential interventions to address health equity for 2 years; staff have recently completed health equity training along with training in population health	**Weaknesses** • What might happen to our role in the broader system if we don't make this change? *Case example*: Program outcomes will continue to reflect significant disparities; staff and community contractors interested in innovative approaches to health equity may become discouraged by the lack of commitment and target action to change outcomes • What knowledge, talent, skills, and/or resources are we lacking to make this change? *Case example*: Some program staff are used to serving individuals vs. working at the population health level; staff from every organizational program involved in the change are not supportive

(continued)

EXHIBIT 3.1 SWOT Tool for Readiness Assessment (*continued*)

EXTERNAL ASPECTS	Opportunities	Threats
	■ What are the broader systems mandates or calls for change in our field? How can we leverage existing momentum? *Case example*: State social movements are demanding health equity; the state has received funding for innovative approaches to health equity	■ Are there changes in our field or broader systems that could threaten our future without this change? *Case example*: Communities experiencing disparities will lose confidence in government to address their issues; systems fragmentation will continue without shared outcomes or collaborative community efforts
	■ What is our unique role to play in the broader system that is calling for change? *Case example*: Historically, the state has served as a natural convener to seed and gain support for innovative approaches around critical health issues, so acting on this issue is consistent with the state's role in the past	■ Are there resource constraints that could make this change difficult to complete? *Case example*: Not all federal funds dedicated to this change are flexible. Federal waivers may be necessary
	■ Is there a need that is not currently being met that we can fill? *Case example*: The need to demonstrate significant improvements in health outcomes for all populations	■ Are there other political priorities that might impede the change? *Case example*: The executive branch is watchful of "government overreach," prizing personal responsibility; the County Commissioners Organization will need to be brought "on board"
	■ Are there other social systems involved in this type of work with whom we might partner to make this change? *Case example*: State Human Services and Medicaid are re-designing data systems that will allow for integrated data collection	■ Are there other social systems involved in this type of work with whom we might end up "competing" if we undertake this change? *Case example*: The State Office of Health Equity will need to "buy in"

After completing the SWOT, debrief by asking yourself or the group these questions:

- What are your main takeaways from this activity?
- How does this change your thinking about the proposed change?
- What do the results indicate about your organization's readiness to undertake the proposed change?
- What are your action steps as a result of this activity?

Box 3.1 Readiness activities for leaders

1. Assess your status as a learning organization
2. Facilitate change conversations
3. Support individual-level readiness assessments, such as the Change Style Indicator® (CSI)
4. Facilitate organizational-level readiness assessments, such as a modified SWOT (strengths, weaknesses, opportunities, threats)

Box 3.1 summarizes how the activities and tools described earlier can be used to enhance readiness.

IMPLEMENTING CHANGE

This section addresses several facets of implementing change: stakeholder engagement to develop/understand shared goals (listening sessions); having a learning mindset (Plan-Do-Check/Study-Act [PDSA]); timing your change and addressing resistance.

The assessment process described can clarify the reasons for seeking change, where the change needs to occur, and how to proceed. For instance, in this chapter's case example, bureau heads may identify which funding streams can be braided and how internal accounting and external reporting would need to change to accomplish this. Once participants have identified the need for change, they often feel an urgency to act. External stakeholders such as funders can also be eager to see demonstrable progress quickly. At this point, it is often actually wise to reduce expectations for speed in order to allow enough time to prepare for the level of adaption significant change will entail. Several months to a year of deep listening to key partners and other stakeholders is often necessary to develop sufficient commitment to common goals and clarity about roles.[8] This process may occur across multiple stages of an action plan timeline.

The time-intensive nature of collaborative capacity building is particularly true of cross-sectoral initiatives such as the community-based funding initiative described in the case example. Often, people assume that they share specific beliefs and goals with others more than they do, especially when they share broader goals. This can lead to painful surprises as collaboration proceeds and partners act on divergent assumptions. Collaboration also necessitates clarity about who can devote the necessary time to moving a change process forward, typically for a number of months.

It is also true that change implementation must inevitably occur before all relevant information is available. To frame this in an admittedly arbitrary way, when leaders feel about 80% ready, it is time to jump in and start making the changes identified as most needed. Then, as implementation proceeds, leaders should monitor both "hard" and "soft" data to track progress and problems and recalibrate plans accordingly. "Hard" data may include financial costs; how much time people are spending on the change process; when milestones are being met relative to plans; and number of people served.

"Soft" data may include participant and other stakeholder enthusiasm or withdrawal, as well as perceptions of initiative success.

The hallmarks of a learning organization[2] can again be used as touchpoints. Applying a learning mindset to change will feel a lot harder in the midst of implementation than in the early days of planning but will be all the more important when the process is the most challenging. One way to improve learning from implementation challenges is to apply quality improvement "Plan-Do-Check/Study-Act" cycles throughout the change initiative. This PDSA approach treats change as a series of incremental experiments, including clarifying goals and strategies, pilot testing, reviewing progress, and incorporating feedback from this review into the next stage of the experiment.[9] As a leader, you should reflect on how you may be resisting your own change efforts, for instance, through controlling processes too tightly rather than creating the conditions for collective change or failing to incorporate the results of incremental experiments.[8]

Significant change prompts resistance, as people brace for associated losses. As noted earlier, anticipating who may resist, how, and why is an important element of assessing change readiness. For instance, in the case example, people responsible for programs losing designated funding when funds are combined are likely to resist this restructuring. People also often resist changes that require them to acquire new skills or substantially change work routines. Resistance may be motivated by personal agendas or may even be well-founded but incompatible with broader goals. In those instances, you may need to reduce some individuals' influence. You may also need to proceed more cautiously or back off some goals if they conflict with powerful stakeholders' priorities.[10] For instance, advocacy groups can lobby with legislatures or agency leadership to block change, and a state's political environment may limit funding or programmatic options.

Resistance to change can be taxing or even ugly. A learning perspective will help maintain distance from the emotional heat of such encounters and distinguish between destructive and potentially constructive resistance. Often the people affected by change have a deep knowledge of related processes. They may also have insights based on prior initiatives or distrust based on past or current mismanagement of change.[11] Actively eliciting concerns, deeply listening, making amends for current or prior breaches of commitment, and sometimes shifting course may lead to fairer and more effective implementation. Some initial skeptics may also "convert" if they see new processes succeed.

Evidence shows that managers often become less committed to systems changes just months before success becomes self-reinforcing.[12] While leaders must be prepared to adapt along the path of change, they must also keep moving forward and communicating confidence when resistance arises and other priorities compete for participants' attention.

CHANGE LEADERSHIP AND MANAGEMENT SKILLS

Once readiness has been assessed and achieved (or sometimes even if those processes are still underway) leaders can also draw on skills from their daily leadership practice when supporting change. Multiple types of skills are useful. "Head skills" correlate clearly with the capacity readiness skills described earlier and include (a) maintaining focus on the end goal by articulating a clear vision of the desired outcome; (b) leading strategic planning processes to document how the vision will be operationalized;

and (c) communicating expectations, progress, roles, and achievements and setbacks. "Heart skills" correlate most closely with the motivational readiness skills described earlier and include (a) building and maintaining trust; (b) communicating transparently; (c) connecting individuals with an emotional anchor for change relevance; and (d) committing to the change over time, holding steady when resistance emerges. This final idea of holding steady can also be thought of as grit. The amount of time devoted to change efforts often far exceeds initial leadership estimates, and strong leaders often display the grit desired to push the change across the finish line when others have given up.

Both "head" and "heart" are reflected in the SWOT analysis for the case example; savvy leaders will utilize this information in crafting their messaging, strategies, and measurements of progress.

Much has been written about change leadership, but the less compelling idea of change *management* is often the unsung hero of successful change initiatives. Some leaders have strong skills in both visioning and the details of execution, but it is more common to see less proficiency in operational management. For example, change leaders may identify policy changes that are necessary to support a particular change. Being able to hand off the task of updating policies to a "change manager" can free you up to continue uncovering innovations and articulating the vision. However, you must clearly delegate the authority for change management and continue to communicate strong support for the mechanics of the change process.

When considering the breadth of skills that are useful to change efforts, you might want to do a quick initial inventory of your own skills for leading change as you embark on a new change initiative. You may then be able to identify other individuals to fill in the gaps as necessary to provide these critical capacities in support of the proposed change.

In some cases, thinking of change leadership and management as the responsibility of a small change mini-team rather than solely an individual effort can help relieve the stress of having to "do it all" when it comes to leading a significant change. Building a mini-change team up front can also provide a sounding board, encouragement, and accountability as the change effort is developed and implemented. Referring back to the case example, a change mini-team could be created with some staff and managers whose programs will be involved in the change, along with someone less directly involved who might bring "fresh eyes" to the process.

NON CYNICAL REALISM

Any change effort requires a healthy dose of non cynical realism. Most professionals have participated in change efforts that have fallen short of their goals and recognize that the good intentions of a few strong leaders are not sufficient to overcome organizational and structural inertia in systems. Leaders can prepare for change by both understanding and communicating the learning, including failures, derived from previous change efforts. Transparency is critical to holding rumors and cynicism at bay, while also fostering a healthy balance between optimism and realism. In all types of change efforts, it is critical for leaders to find thought partners within and sometimes beyond their change team who can honestly and carefully assess progress together and redirect efforts as necessary.

Another key aspect of non cynical realism is flexibility. Strong change leaders recognize, articulate, and embrace the fact that change may not follow a direct path, and indeed the end results may not even resemble the early stated goals of the process. As system participants begin to engage deeply in the change process, they will bring their own insights, learning, and experiences to the work. As a result, the intermediate goals may change. Efforts may shift from an expected "low hanging fruit" effort to an entirely different sector or area of change. A critical role of change leaders is to help the group maintain a focus on the larger goal while still supporting and facilitating logical shifts in the path along the way. Change efforts, especially those in cross-sector systems, always take on a life of their own in response to the context in which they unfold.

Change sponsors can be allies in this area. Sponsors such as foundations and other funders often provide incentives (i.e., grant funding, unifying frameworks, convening of stakeholders) to advance their vision of systems change for a particular community or issue. Political leaders such as governors can also serve as a unifying force for systems change. In your work, you may be able to call upon relevant change sponsors to reinforce a broad vision as a "rallying cry," spurring continued work and progress. Change sponsors may also be enlisted to provide "cover" for organizational leaders when resistance emerges or turf battles arise.

The tips for implementing change described earlier are synthesized in Box 3.2.

Box 3.2 Tips for implementing change

1. Manage expectations
2. Listen and learn
3. Jump in
4. Keep learning
5. Adapt and persist
6. Partner with sponsors

In sum, readiness for change is one phase of systems change, and the elements of readiness can be described as $R = MC^2$, where **Readiness** = **M**otivation x general organizational **C**apacity and specific **C**apacity to undertake the change under consideration. As elsewhere in this book, this chapter builds on the premise that change is iterative.

Figure 3.1 summarizes the foundational readiness activities described in this chapter: hallmarks of learning organizations, change conversations, and readiness assessments. Organizations that support personal mastery, team learning, shared vision, systems thinking, and clear mental models have a readiness advantage. However, even when your change context is not strong in all of these hallmarks of learning organizations, you can use informal change conversations to assess readiness for systems change and gauge where more preparation is necessary. Such conversations involve intentionally exploring the who, what, when, why, where, and how of any potential change.

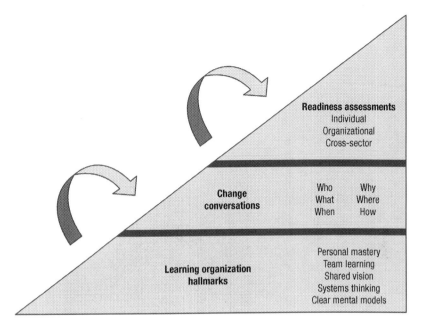

Figure 3.1 Foundational readiness activities.

More formal readiness assessments can also help you understand where the "pain points" of change are most likely to emerge. Like learning organization hallmarks and the takeaways that emerge from change conversations, formal readiness assessments advance readiness through clarifying and sharing understanding. In turn, these conversations can yield ideas about where to intervene to enhance readiness. The CSI is one option for individuals to explore their own personal readiness. A modified SWOT can be used to identify organizational facilitators and barriers for alternative potential changes.

Leaders should use their own "head" and "heart" skills to advance readiness for systems change by reducing stakeholders' expectations for swift progress while also preparing to proceed before feeling fully ready, approaching the change with non cynical realism, using small tests of change to test the waters and enhance buy-in, preparing for and managing resistance, and ensuring enough attention to both the broader leadership vision and the myriad details of change management.

CHAPTER SUMMARY

Public health change is complex, is vitally important, and often occurs in the context of significant constraints. The ideas and tools in this chapter can help you improve your organization's readiness to undertake and implement change at the individual, organizational, and systems levels. Leaders can help ensure readiness by applying an understanding of systems dynamics, clarifying goals, and using formal or informal readiness assessments. We shared a readiness formula and three tools to help leaders get teams ready for change and also offered some additional guidance about resistance and timing.

Key Messages

- Habits of self-assessment, skills in collective learning, and a systems orientation can improve prospects for successful change.
- Using change conversations can set the stage for change in your organization. These conversations can be used in conjunction with more formal readiness assessments.
- Readiness assessments are important and should be completed prior to implementation of any significant change initiative.

Tips

- First, understand your own change leadership (and management) strengths and your own change style preference.
- Next, clarify what change may be needed, why, and how. Be explicit: Do not assume common goals, beliefs, or mental models.
- Assessing readiness for change can be relatively simple; however, the importance of such assessments and change conversations cannot be over emphasized.
- Change initiatives frequently require more time and effort than originally intended, especially for communicating sufficiently with a range of stakeholders.
- Resistance to change is normal and while it can be fierce, it can also improve the implementation plan by surfacing barriers and gaps. Addressing these can enhance the success of the change initiative and the credibility of change leaders.

Supplemental Resources

- Learning Organizations: https://elearningindustry.com/key-traits-learning -organizations
- Change Styles: https://elearningindustry.com/key-traits-learning-organizations; www.leadershipiq.com/blogs/leadershipiq/86843777-quiz-whats-your-style-of -change-management
- Change Style Indicator® (CSI®): https://alievo.com/our-services/assessment-tools /change-style-indicator/?lang=en
- SWOT Analyses: www.mindtools.com/pages/article/newTMC_05.htm

REFERENCES

1. Lewin K. Frontiers in group dynamics: concepts, method, and reality in social science. *Hum Relat*. 1947;1(1):5–41. doi:10.1177/001872674700100103.
2. Scaccia JP, Cook BS, Lamont A, et al. A practical implementation science heuristic for organizational readiness: R= MC^2. *J Commun Psychol*. 2015;43(4):484–501. doi:10.1002/jcop.21698.
3. Blair JD, Whitehead C. Too many on the seesaw: stakeholder diagnosis and management for hospitals. *Hosp Health Serv Admin*. 1988;33(2):153–166. PMID: 10302490.
4. Peters DH. The application of systems thinking in health: why use systems thinking? *Health Res Policy Syst*. 2014;12(1):1–6. doi:10.1186/1478-4505-12-51.
5. Smith PAC. Action learning and reflective practice in project environments that are related to leadership development. *Manage Learn*. 2001;32(1):31–48. doi:10.1177/1350507601321003.
6. Learned A, Christensen C, Andrews R, et al. *Business Policy: Text and Cases*. Irwin; 1965.
7. Bryson JM. *Strategic Planning for Public and Nonprofit Organizations: A Guide to Strengthening and Sustaining Organizational Achievement*. John Wiley & Sons; 2018.
8. Senge P, Hamilton H, Kania J. The dawn of system leadership. *Stanf Soc Innov Rev*. 2015;13(1):27–33. doi:10.48558/YTE7-XT62.
9. Moen R, Norman C. *Evolution of the PDCA Cycle*. Citeseer; 2006.
10. Lozeau D, Langley A, Denis J-L. The corruption of managerial techniques by organizations. *Hum Relat*. 2002;55(5):537–564. doi:10.1177/0018726702055005427.
11. Ford JD, Ford LW, D'Amelio A. Resistance to change: the rest of the story. *Acad Manage Rev*. 2008;33(2):362–377. doi:10.2307/20159402.
12. Repenning NP. A simulation-based approach to understanding the dynamics of innovation implementation. *Org Sci*. 2003;13(2):109–127. doi:10.1287/orsc.13.2.109.535.

The Levels and Success Practices for Systems Change in Public Health

II

4

Personal Leadership: The Requirement to Show Up Authentically to Advance Systems Change

Kristina Y. Risley and Renée Branch Canady

CHAPTER OBJECTIVES

By the end of this chapter, the practitioner will be able to:

- Define personal leadership and the role it plays in systems change.
- Identify critical evidence-based practices to develop oneself as a leader.
- Engage in exercises to grow one's leadership capacity.
- Reflect on leadership strengths and gaps.

INTRODUCTION

Pick a side. You are either awake or asleep; speaking or listening; sitting or standing; certain or unsure. Similarly, you are either leading or following. While both roles are needed, there is little room to straddle the leadership fence. Every leadership opportunity that you chose to forego is a missed opportunity to be a part of something important and vital. The importance and vitality of leadership is not always measured by scope and scale. The impact of your actions may influence one person, one department, one city, one state, or one nation. Similarly, your actions may influence numerous people, several departments, and multiple cities, states, and nations. Most importantly, within those settings are systems, large and small, where the impact of your actions can be felt.

To lead systems change that improves the effectiveness and efficiency of the work you do with others in your organization and that ultimately sets you up to engage in work with diverse stakeholders that improves public health, it is imperative that you have a lifelong focus on leadership development. You can think of leadership development at multiple levels, including the personal, interpersonal, team, organizational, and systems levels. At each of these levels, there are practices that support ongoing development. At the personal level, leadership development helps you gain clarity about who you are and what you stand for as a leader and how you think and act differently and similarly than your colleagues and your stakeholder partners. As a result, you not only have the capacity to lead through your knowledge and skills but also through your presence, empathy, and compassion. This combination of leadership skills helps to better guide the efforts you undertake in your agency and helps you better align, coordinate, and/or collaborate your efforts to achieve maximum beneficial change in your community's health.

Your leadership is more important today than ever. This is a unique time in history distinguished by a worldwide pandemic and a call to end racism. Many of us are reflecting on the dire importance of public health leadership. As with past pandemics, coronavirus disease (COVID) will eventually resolve or dampen; the commitment to ending racism so that all people have access to whole health is stronger than ever and becoming a more pointed focus. It is important that peoples' opinions of public health be based on more than a worldwide pandemic. Similarly, the public's understanding of public health leaders must also be deeper than a singular event. This moment in time allows us to demonstrate who we are as public health leaders, but it is not the genesis of who we are as public health leaders—that genesis is steeped in who we are, how we are, and why each of us chose this vital profession.

This chapter invites you to begin, refine, and/or strengthen your commitment to a leadership journey and public health, starting with the most important component—yourself! As such, this chapter focuses on critical personal leadership characteristics and practices to assist you on this journey. It is a journey that will move you beyond public health expert and into the role of public health leader.

PERSONAL LEADERSHIP

What Is Personal Leadership?

Peter Senge, a leading systems scientist, scholar, and author of *The Fifth Discipline: The Art & Practice of the Learning Organization*,[1] coined the term "personal mastery" as a core discipline for individuals who desire to thrive in their work and for organizations that desire to harness the brilliant ideas of their employees. Personal mastery focuses on your own personal growth and development. It becomes a discipline when you make a lifelong commitment to develop yourself. Such a commitment involves seeing your current reality with increasing clarity and honesty, clarifying what matters to you, and aligning your life and work with what matters most to you. In the context of our busy and complex lives, it is so easy to forget who we are and what matters most.

Personal mastery as part of systems change is critical for organizations that desire to stay on the leading edge of public health. Organizations can only respond to changing public health needs when the individuals in the organizations learn and grow.

Personal mastery becomes personal leadership when you take action, based on an understanding of your growth and development, to lead the change you want to see in the world. Not only are you committed to being a competent and skilled public health technical or subject matter expert, but you are also dedicated to work that aligns with your growth and development.[2] You align your work and values, and you feel compelled to develop the leadership competencies and skills needed to create vision, innovative strategies, and tactics that improve the conditions in which all people have the opportunity to be healthy.

For example, as a result of the COVID-19 pandemic, many of you became clearer and more vocal about how you value anti-racism and equity. You recognize that this value aligns with who you are as a person and your work in public health. You experience racism as a public health problem, and you are committed to dismantling the systems that keep institutional racism in place. Many of your places of employment took a stand on this issue by preparing anti-racism statements that call for us all to once and for all address this horrible problem. Many places of employment have also taken immediate action by assessing and changing internal policies, practices, and procedures designed to support equitable workplaces. Further, the field acknowledges equity as essential work and included it as the most important of the 10 Essential Public Health Services.[3] When your personal values align with the values of your place of employment and the work more broadly addressed in the public health field, there is greater incentive for you to express your personal leadership. This can result in leadership opportunities coming your way as well as you taking on more leadership in this and other areas of alignment.

Adult Development Theory and Personal Leadership

Adult development theory provides a useful foundation to think about how personal leadership development may become of interest and manifest in you. It highlights that even as adults you can continue to grow, develop, and adapt. Strong leaders must be willing to grow, develop, and adapt. As you develop from an adolescent into an adult, you may find yourself moving from the need to live your life according to external or societal expectations to creating your life and work by looking inside yourself to explore the difference you want to make in the world, effectively designing and leading your own life. It is from this internal place that you have the potential to create a true and meaningful vision for your work and life as well as the steps to lead you toward your own north star versus the north star someone else may think is right or best for you.

Robert Kegan's five-stage constructive developmental theory[4] is one of many that highlight the adult developmental process. The stages of development include the (a) impulsive mind (early childhood); (b) imperial mind (adolescence); (c) socialized mind (late teens through 20s; just over half of all adults are estimated to reach this stage of development); (d) self-authoring mind; and (e) self-transforming mind (fewer than 1% of adults). The later stages of development, self-authoring and self-transforming, generally begin in your 30s and can continue through the remainder of your life, providing you with a canvas on which to define (or refine) who you are and the change you want to lead in the world. Notably, it is estimated that fewer than half of all adults reach the self-authoring mind stage of development and less than 1% of adults reach the self-transforming mind stage of development.

This theory also helps us to see how it is possible for each of us to see and experience the world differently. Because of the unique ways that people develop, we live in a world with multiple and often contradictory ways of framing and expressing values. This complexity of values creates challenges for how we will or will not work together to create systems change to improve community health. When we are aware of this reality, we can engage practices to help us see who we are, how we are similar and different from others, and how we might align to improve community health even when we have very different histories, beliefs, and strategies.

Personal Leadership and Emotional and Social Intelligence

As your capacity to see yourself and others more clearly expands, your emotional and social intelligence improves. Being an emotionally intelligent leader means that you know yourself deeply; you can create a vision for your life and work. In addition, you can manage the wide range of emotions you experience, getting out of your own way and in alignment with your highest potential for the sake of the greater good.

Being a socially intelligent leader means that you have empathy and compassion; you know how to meet others where they are in order to inspire and bring out the best in their leadership and work. Leaders with emotional and social intelligence communicate effectively and manage conflict when it arises or are willing to stay in the conversation when communication goes awry. They work successfully in collaboration with others even when challenges arise. You can develop explicit emotional and social intelligence competencies.

Specific emotional intelligence (EI) competencies include self-awareness, self-assessment, self-confidence, self-control, transparency, adaptability, achievement, initiative, and optimism.[5] Specific social intelligence competencies (SI) include empathy, organizational awareness, service, inspiration, influence, developing others, change catalyst, conflict management, and teamwork/collaboration.[5] Developing competency in these critical leadership areas enhances your ability to work with diverse stakeholders to achieve shared goals. These are necessary competencies above and beyond your technical skills or subject matter expertise; they will take you further faster in your career and they will help you be a more effective leader than those without these competencies.

With these competencies squarely grounded in your leadership, you have the increased internal capacity to better understand your own and other's perceptions of reality and create the systems changes needed to support more equitable and healthier communities. These competencies help you to create the space that makes it possible for you to step into new opportunities to improve the likelihood that together you can create a shared future that is equitable for all.

Aligning Personal Leadership and Systems Change in Public Health

Kegan's developmental theory provides a framework for reflection and assessment that must be juxtaposed with our personal leadership in the broader context of our public health practice. The Six Conditions of Systems Change[6] provides an important and complementary frame to Kegan's framework and for situating ourselves as public health systems leaders. Among the six conditions presented in the model, three stand out as especially salient for personal leadership considerations: (a) mental models, (b) relationships and connections, and (c) power dynamics.

Mental models are defined as "deeply held beliefs and assumptions and taken-for-granted ways of operating that influence how we think, what we do, and how we talk."[6(p4)] Deeply held beliefs evolve during the stage described by Kegan as the socialized mind. As such, aligning personal leadership with systems change may require a level of intentionality that allows us to "unlearn" deeply learned models, especially if they lend themselves to the greater benefit of one group over another. Mental models can influence how we engage others, and more importantly, are egocentrically aligned. Our mental models make sense to us and they establish our worldview. Systems change by its very nature presumes the need for modification and variation. Leaders must strive to make the invisible visible as they assess the relevance of their personal mental models to a broader worldview.

Relationships and connections provide the vehicle for action. Whether advancing collective impact or strategizing to engage a stakeholder who holds a contrary point of view, leaders must be mindful of which authentic relationships to leverage and when. Dr. Ron David says, "relationships are primary; all else is derivative."[7] Relationships allow you to advance change, make decisions, apply concepts, and execute practices. With the public as the primary focus of our field, the collective nature of the profession is underscored. Public health is "what we do together to assure [sic] the health of the public"[8]—in other words, what we do in relationships to ensure the health of the public.

The volume of relationships determines your reach and whom you engage. The nature of relationships underscores how you engage. What is the span of your influence, the reach of your relationships? The nature of your relationships enables trust and continuity. What is the quality of your relationships? Equally, the nature of your relationships establishes their longevity. How you listen and hear the needs of others relative to your own priorities and agenda will guarantee that relationships persist for the next issue. How you engage becomes the foundation for building trust and recognizing that trust is earned, not given.

Relationships and connections are also integrally tied to power dynamics. Building relationships with individuals who hold decision-making authority and influence as well as recognizing your own authority and influence, regardless of your placement in your organization, build power. Understanding power as the ability to implement change to meet your needs or the needs of others allows you to visualize and implement broad change in immediate areas of influence and across systems. Relationships are a precious leadership resource in which to invest and protect. Power as a consequence is not to be feared or avoided but to be built and intentionally applied to the unique responsibilities of public health.

The effective integration of mental models, relationships and connections, and power dynamics requires us to integrate the cognitive and the affective—what we know and what we feel. Leading with head and heart keeps us in a place of authenticity. For public health leaders to enter the controversy that so often pervades our field and shift stagnant mental models, we must utilize flexibility, curiosity, persistence, boldness, and risk taking. As seen in the lives of John Snow, considered the founder of epidemiology, and Lillian Wald, considered the founder of public health nursing, pursuing purpose and rejecting the status quo allowed them to advance significant systems change. For example, Dr. John Snow is attributed with identifying the Broad Street pump as the source of the 1854 cholera outbreak in London.[9] As a physician, he could have simply treated the patients with this disease but he used his privilege and extended his role beyond that of the customary physician to advocate and apply his knowledge to resolve a public health problem. Similarly, Lillian Wald, who was also a woman of privilege and means, upon completion of her nursing training, began working to create a more just society, focusing her attention on immigrant families and those living in poverty. Rather than practicing her profession in the customary manner for the time, she introduced the innovative idea of nurses going to patients in their homes, thus giving rise to the Visiting Nurse Service.[10] Furthermore, her advocacy for those in poverty pushed her to coin the now common term "public health nurse," gathering like-minded partners to advance change. These early innovative ideas of Snow and Wald, birthed by the demonstration of courageous leadership, ultimately changed systems and became common practice.

The Proving Ground of Personal Leadership in Public Health

Today, the field of public health is more focused on personal leadership development than at any other time in history. It is increasingly presented on and workshopped at conferences. It is integrated into foundational workforce efforts, including the public health core competencies, the National Consortium for Public Health Workforce Development strategic skills, workforce development plans, and leadership programs. It is implicit in the Certified Public Health Domains and appropriate for inclusion in workforce development plans described in the Public Health Accreditation Board's Standards and Measures. (Domain 8: Maintain a Competent Public Health).[11]

Since 2014, the Health Resources and Services Administration's (HRSA) Maternal and Child Health Bureau (MCHB) has funded the National Maternal and Child Health Workforce Center, which also provides training, consultation, and coaching to, in part, help public health leaders develop their personal leadership. The MCHB defines personal leadership as self-reflection or the "process of assessing the impact of personal values, beliefs, communication styles, cultural influences, and experiences on personal and professional leadership."[12] This work is not singular to MCHB; increasingly, practitioners across the field have access to the practices and resources they need to become courageous and bold systems change leaders.

Here we highlight specific practices for developing personal leadership. These practices can be divided into three buckets, including: (a) defining your leadership, (b) growing yourself as a leader, and (c) sustaining your leadership. While you may be looking for tools, let us offer a reframe. Abraham Maslow said, "I suppose it is tempting, if the only tool you have is a hammer, to treat everything as if it were a nail."[13] Too often, public health leaders fail to see themselves as the most important tool in their toolbox; you are the tool. As such, we encourage you to avoid the typical clamoring for tools as is so common among public health practitioners. Instead, let's begin by exploring grounding practices.

More specifically, we begin by looking at how you ground yourself as a leader. We focus on grounding practices to (a) assess your mental models, (b) articulate your values, (c) identify your life purpose, and (d) establish a vision for your work in public health. Next, we look at how you grow as a leader, focusing on practices to (a) identify your leadership strengths and (b) assess your emotional and social intelligence. Finally, we look at how to sustain your leadership as well as lead with equanimity by staying in tune with yourself and others through a mindfulness practice. With these practices, you can begin your journey to serve as a beacon of light guiding the way toward a more compassionate and forward-thinking field of public health and society that values all people equitably.

HOW DO I GROUND MYSELF AS A LEADER?

Most of us, when asked the proverbial question, "What do you want to be when you grow up?" did not reply "a public health professional," and we certainly did not reply "a public health leader." Many of us in the public health workforce did not seek out this profession; rather, the profession found us. In fact, only 17% of the public health workforce holds a degree in public health, at any level.[14] Efforts such as the National Public Health Week, organized for over 25 years by the American Public Health Association, seek to increase the public's understanding of this vital profession. However, confusion over the distinctions between healthcare, community health, and public health remains common. Were it not for the sweeping impact of the coronavirus pandemic, little attention would currently be afforded to the public health field. Intriguingly, circuitous journeys bring professionals to the field and indirect paths raise public knowledge of the profession. These convoluted contexts are indicative of the dire need for leadership and pose important opportunities for public health leaders.

In addition to the limited formal education of public health professionals and limited public understanding of the profession (pre-COVID), those with knowledge of public health face numerous challenges. Koh and Jacobson[15] illuminate the complexity and huge scale of public health problems. They also underscore the complexity of public health problems and the extended investment of time needed to resolve them. We see these characteristics play out in the COVID pandemic. Numerous stakeholders have raised diverse and often conflicting perspectives. Despite our efforts to apply customary rapid response initiatives often used in public health emergencies, the pace of reversing a worldwide pandemic is never rapid enough for public stakeholders or elected officials. Another example is the call for racism to be viewed as a public health crisis. Racism is a systemic problem, it affects everyone, and it is the cause of the disparities in health outcomes between White people and Black, Indigenous, and other people of color.

Such characteristics seen in the intransigent examples of a pandemic of a novel virus and the "pandemic" of racism and social unrest clearly demand that we acknowledge our mental models, values, purpose, and public health vision. They also demand that we identify our leadership strengths; assess our emotional and social intelligence; and lead with courage, boldness, and equanimity. In the following, we describe practices to help you grow in each of these critical aspects of personal leadership.

Exercise 1: Mental Models

As stated earlier in the chapter, mental models have been described as "habits of thought—deeply held beliefs and assumptions and taken-for-granted ways of operating that influence how we think, what we do, and how we talk."[6(p4)] While seemingly complex, our focus on mental models simply requires us to recognize that they exist. There are worldviews, underlying assumptions, and mental frameworks that float below the surface of our thinking. As leaders, we must pause and think about our thinking! What are the implicit factors that are shaping our opinions and even our preferences? What are the unspoken assumptions and deeply held beliefs that inform our thinking? Examples of deeply held beliefs include the ideas that leaders have the final say, leaders set the priorities, and leaders hold elevated positions. The following is a set of questions to consider to shed light on your mental models. These are not easy questions to answer; however, they will uncover where you might be holding yourself back as a leader and how you might limit the desired impact in your professional relationships and partnerships.

1.   What are the unspoken factors that shape your thinking about—?
2.   What aspects of culture and climate influence your thinking about—?
3.   What inherited beliefs might be influencing your efforts and decision-making about—?
4.   Is my response a consequence of present information or is it overly informed by my past personal experiences?
5.   Has this practice of—changed in the past 5 to 10 years or is it a relic of conditions that no longer exist?

Exercise 2: Values Clarification

Leadership researchers James Kouzes and Barry Posner have found in their studies that leaders at their peak engage in a handful of exemplary leadership practices, including: (a) model the way, (b) inspire a shared vision, (c) challenge the process, (d) enable others to act, and (e) encourage the heart.[16] A key practice in "model the way" is to clarify your values. Below we provide you with a process to help you articulate your values. The prompts provided are inspired by one of the author's coaching (Risley) training with the Co-Active Institute that will help you articulate your values.[17] Examples can come from your personal or professional life. Each prompt will help you surface rich information about what drives you. In Table 4.1, you will find values clarification prompts. Read the prompts and then engage in the steps that follow.

TABLE 4.1 Prompts for Values Clarification	
PROMPT #	**PROMPT DESCRIPTION**
1	Imagine a peak moment in your life. A moment in time when all was right in your world! Some people refer to this as "being in the flow." You could do no wrong and no one could do you any wrong. When was this moment and what was happening? Who was involved? What were you doing? When did this occur? Where did this occur? Why this moment?
2	Name something that makes your mind chatter. Often, there is one or more values that lies beneath that is being stepped on or disrespected by others.
3	Identify a hobby—why do you spend time engaging with this hobby?
4	Identify a person you admire—what about this person do you admire and why?
5	What do you long for in your life? Why?

Now that you have read the prompts, engage the following steps to clarify your values.

1. Select one of the prompts in Table 4.1.
2. In as much detail as possible, journal in a paper or electronic notebook about your experience with the prompt.
3. Identify the values that emerge from your journaling.
4. String together similar words and phrases until you have three to five words or phrases that articulate the fullness of each value. Tip: *Do not aim for perfection. Instead, let the words or phrases be a true reflection of who you are.* An example of a value that includes a string of words and phrases might be: *Freedom/Aliveness/ Anything is possible/Adventure/Seize the moment.* This value is based on a peak moment experience of sitting by Lake Michigan on a beautiful summer day.
5. On a scale of 1 to 10, rate each value as to how much you are living that value in your life. Reflect on what your life might look like if that number were higher.
6. If a number is uncomfortably low, consider action steps that may increase the number.

It is likely that each prompt will harvest more than one value. Each prompt can also be repeated with a different example to identify new values. Make it your goal to identify 10 core values. For a different, more linear approach to identify values, please see the Moral Core exercise included in the book *Resonant Leadership.*[18] This tool may be particularly helpful in preparation for articulating team values discussed in Chapter 7.

Exercise 3: Life Purpose

In the exemplary practice called "inspire a shared vision," Kouzes and Posner write about the importance of finding a common purpose.[11] Knowing your life purpose can help you rally around a common shared purpose. Please note that life purpose means

TABLE 4.2 Life Purpose Scenarios	
SCENARIO 1	**SCENARIO 2**
Imagine you and others are standing in an audience waiting for a talk to begin. On the stage is a wiser version of yourself at some point in the future, your future-self. Your future-self begins to speak and you and the others in the audience are inspired. All of you have been changed forever. Your future self had a profound impact on you, and you will change the way you approach your life and work forever. What was the impact your future-self had on you and others in the audience? How were you and the others transformed? What was the nature of your future-self to have this profound impact?	You have been chosen to design a new community that benefits all its members. You have all the power and resources you need to make this an ideal place for all. When you get started, what is it that you are going to make happen? What is the impact you will have? Imagine your kick-off to the new community. You want people to know what you envision. What is the vision you share with them?

different things to different people and nothing whatsoever to other people. The following is an exercise to help you articulate your life purpose. Take this exercise and use it as is or adapt to fit your own needs; this includes adapting the language of "life purpose" as needed. Tip: *Do not aim for perfection. Aim for good enough. A life purpose can evolve and change over time with experience, knowledge, and wisdom.* In this exercise, you will read two life purpose scenarios (see Table 4.2) and then complete the set of action steps that follow. These scenarios and the metaphor process described in Life Purpose Step Five below are included as part of the co-active coach training provided through the Co-Active Institute and also included in the Co-Active Coaching book.[12] If you prefer, you can record yourself reading these scenarios aloud and then listen to the recordings as you guide yourself through the questions in each scenario and the steps below.

Life Purpose Steps

1. Select a scenario from Table 4.2 and read it.
2. In as much detail as possible, journal in a paper or electronic notebook about your experience with the scenario.
3. Identify the themes you notice in the scenario.
4. Repeat steps 1 to 3 with the other scenario. Once you have journaled about each scenario, identify your themes across the two scenarios. Tip: *Do not aim for perfection. Handle the exercise lightly. Your life purpose can take shape and evolve over time. Instead, let the words or phrases be a true reflection of who you are.*
5. Create a metaphor about your life purpose based on the themes you identified. The metaphor should take the form of: I am the _____(metaphor) so that people _____(impact). Examples of a life purpose statement are *I am the lighthouse that guides people to an equitable future* or *I am the truth that reminds people to keep challenging the status quo.* Tip: If you are having trouble with the metaphor/impact concept, create whatever statement works best for you. An example of this is *I help people connect to self, others, and something greater.*

Once you have completed this exercise, using a scale of 1 to 10, reflect on how much you are living your life on purpose (professionally, personally, overall).

Exercise 4: Public Health Vision

Now that you have completed the mental models, values clarification, and life purpose exercises, you can begin to articulate your public health vision statement. Reflecting on your responses to these three exercises, how might you craft this statement? As an example, the life purpose statement *I help connect people with self, others, and something greater* can translate into the public health vision statement *Leadership development at the individual, team, organizational, and systems levels results in alive and engaged learning and growth and unanticipated innovations in public health scholarship and practice.* This exercise takes time and creativity to complete. Do not be afraid to throw your thoughts on paper. They will evolve and take shape over time. Tip: *Let the statement evolve over time. Print your life purpose and public health vision statements and place them in a location where you see them every day.* Can you practice using these statements to help guide your day-to-day decision-making? If an opportunity or task does not align with either statement or your values, why or how might you consider saying no to the opportunity?

HOW DO I GROW MYSELF AS A LEADER?

Over the decades, there has been an increasing focus on the role of strengths and emotional and social intelligence in leadership development. This is particularly true for the private sector workforce. However, these aspects of leadership development are critical for public health practitioners. In this section of the chapter, we focus on practices to help you grow as a leader by identifying your leadership strengths and assessing your emotional and social intelligence. A focus on strengths is different from performance management, in which a primary strategy is to identify performance gaps and recommended strategies to remedy them. By identifying and building on your strengths, you can develop a strengths-based leadership style that is aligned with your natural talents. It is easier to develop natural talents into strengths than it is to improve upon innate weaknesses.

A focus on emotional and social intelligence is often referred to as developing soft leadership skills; however, these skills are complex because they involve interacting with other human beings. These skills can be continually developed over time and generally set good leaders apart from great leaders. If you want to excel as a leader, focus on developing your emotional and social intelligence. As stated earlier in this chapter, EI is centered on the development of self-focused competencies, including being able to reflect on yourself as a leader (i.e., who you are, what you stand for, your confidence, your ability to self-assess both strengths and challenges). The other component of EI—SI—includes other-focused competencies that include having empathy and compassion as well as the fortitude to work through conflicts and challenges as they arise for the sake of the greater good.

Developing EI and SI is not for the faint of heart. It is much more straightforward to develop yourself as a subject matter expert than it is to dive deep into yourself to find out what makes you a unique and influential leader who others are willing to partner with and follow. The following are exercises to assist you in identifying your leadership strengths and an exercise to assess your EI and SI.

Exercise 1: Leadership Strengths

In this exercise, we highlight a formal assessment tool that has been used by many public health practitioners to help staff and teams begin to build a strengths-based leadership culture. The Gallup Organization's Clifton Strengths Assessment,[19] formally called Clifton StrengthsFinder™, is an online self-assessment that you can use to identify your top five of 34 natural leadership talents/themes. When developed over time, your talents/themes become your leadership strengths. These strengths are plotted into four unique leadership domains: (a) executing, (b) influencing, (c) relationship building, and (d) strategic thinking. These domains provide clarity and explicit language to help you articulate your natural leadership style.

Research indicates that individuals who know and use their strengths are more engaged and productive at work and are generally happier and healthier. Additionally, this body of work provides important information about how to use your strengths so that others want to follow you. For more information, visit Gallup's website or read *Strengths-Based Leadership: Great Leaders, Teams, and Why People Follow*,[19] which includes a unique code for you to self-administer the online assessment.

Exercise 2: Emotional and Social Intelligence

In this exercise, we encourage you to consider completing the EI assessment included in the book *Emotional Intelligence 2.0*.[20] Like *Strengths-Based Leadership*,[19] this book also includes a unique link to complete an online assessment. This assessment provides you with a report about your EI in four competencies: (a) self-awareness, (b) self-management, (c) social awareness, and (d) relationship management. You receive an overall EI score, and scores in each of the four competency areas. Additionally, you receive strategies for how to increase these scores.

HOW DO I RENEW AND SUSTAIN MYSELF AS A LEADER?

In their book *Resonant Leadership*,[18] Richard Boyatzis and Annie McKee coined the phrase Sacrifice Syndrome. You may find yourself in the Sacrifice Syndrome when you are in crisis mode and experiencing any number of threats. When you are in the Sacrifice Syndrome, it means that you are out of tune or dissonant with yourself; this causes you to feel ineffective as a leader. For example, during the COVID-19 pandemic, public health practitioners around the country questioned their effectiveness as leaders. The long-term crisis and response that involved testing, contact tracing, vaccine distribution, and planning strategies to address COVID-19 variants was and continues to be a challenge. Serving in the long-term crisis mode that a pandemic requires made many feel out of tune with themselves and others, causing them to feel ineffective as leaders.

There are evidence-based practices to renew yourself so that you maintain your effectiveness as a leader, including meaningful relationships with others. These include: (a) mindfulness, (b) hope, and (c) compassion.[15] While these are not meant to be quick fixes or particularly easy to implement during a crisis, even one step in the direction of mindfulness, hope, and/or compassion is likely to help you feel that you have some agency over your life and work. This sense of agency will improve over time and with a disciplined practice.

We focus specifically on the establishment of a mindfulness practice because it serves as the foundation for resonant leadership so that you can get and stay in tune with yourselves and others. To learn more about developing hope and compassion, please consider reading the book *Resonant Leadership*[18] referenced earlier.

Exercise 1: Foundational Mindfulness Practice

Boyatzis and McKee define mindfulness as having the capacity to be aware of everything that is going on inside of you as well as outside of you. This means that at any given moment, you are aware of the state of your body, mind, heart, and spirit, and you also are aware of what is going on in your surroundings and with other people. Jon Kabat-Zinn, a leading expert in mindfulness, defines mindfulness as "awareness that arises through paying attention, on purpose, in the present moment, non-judgmentally."[21] Tara Brach, a well-known mindfulness teacher, defines mindfulness as "a way of paying attention moment-to-moment to what's happening within and around us without judgment."[22]

A simple practice goes a long way in establishing the foundation for being more present in your life and work. Here we provide a foundational mindfulness practice.

1. Find a quiet place where you can sit comfortably, uninterrupted, and with an upright spine. Note: If your body hurts, you will meditate on your pain. You do not want to meditate on your pain. You want to use your meditation as a way to improve your attention or awareness.
2. Close your eyes. Bring your attention to your breath. Breathe in slowly to the count of four and exhale slowly to the count of four.
3. When thoughts, feelings, or sensations arise, and they will, imagine them floating by like a cloud in the sky.
4. Focus all your attention on your breath and know that you are so much more than your thoughts and feelings; please do not hold yourself small as a result of negative thoughts and feelings that stream through your mind.

Over time and with practice, this exercise will help you develop the skill of presence so that you are increasingly agile in your ability to deal with the day-to-day pressures that come your way at work. If practiced with some degree of discipline, this exercise gives you access to a deeper well of ideas, including those that may allow you to have a greater impact in your public health work.

This practice takes time to cultivate, and you may not see immediate results; however, if you make this practice a discipline you will see results over time. In my personal experience (Risley), it is the one practice that serves as the foundation for all the great things that have emerged over the course of my life and my saving grace, particularly in challenging and painful times both personally and professionally.

Begin practicing this exercise with 5 minutes per session. Early morning while it is quiet and still outside helps to facilitate the best experience; however, do what works best for you. When this feels easy, increase your minutes. Advanced mindfulness practitioners sit for up to an hour at a time and some more than this. Adding in a few moments of journaling at the end of your session, focused on what you know or think is different at the end of your practice, can serve to provide novel insights about your work and life. Tip: *Do not judge your meditation experience. All meditation experiences are valuable even when they feel like they were not successful.*

Mindfulness helps you develop leadership presence. It also serves as a foundation and discipline to support all the practices provided in this chapter. And it provides the needed space to do the inner work necessary to support your work related to health equity and racial justice. As you continue to educate folks about racism as a public health challenge that needs population-based strategies in order to achieve health and well-being for all, it is important to bring awareness to your personal relationship with racism and racial justice. Rhonda Magee, who wrote the book called *The Inner Work of Racial Justice: Healing Ourselves and Transforming Our Communities Through Mindfulness,*[23] provides a useful framework for how to apply mindfulness to our racial justice leadership.

CHAPTER SUMMARY

In this chapter, we highlighted the reality that you are either leading or following. Every leadership opportunity that you choose to forego is a missed opportunity to be part of something important and vital. Your leadership may influence one person, one department, one city, one state, or one nation.

To lead systems change, it is imperative that you have a lifelong focus on leadership development. Leadership development at the personal level helps you gain clarity about who you are and what you stand for as a leader as well as how you think and act differently and similarly than your colleagues and stakeholder partners. By refining and/or strengthening your commitment to your personal leadership journey, you can move beyond public health subject matter expert to public health leader.

Key Messages

- Personal leadership is the process of making a lifelong commitment to grow and develop yourself as a leader.
- Personal leadership development includes seeing your current reality with increasing clarity and honesty, clarifying what matters to you, and aligning your life and work around what matters. Organizations can only respond to changing public health needs when the individuals in the organizations learn and grow.
- There are several useful practices you can engage in to help you develop your personal leadership.

Tips

- Identify and explore the mental models or worldviews, underlying assumptions, and mental frameworks that determine how you see the world. Recognize that each of us has a unique set of mental models based on our life experiences.
- Clarify the values that you rely on to guide your life and work. Look at how the choices you have made in your life align with these values.
- Articulate your life purpose and look for how your purpose informs your vision for public health. Articulate your vision for public health and let that vision help guide your decision-making.
- Identify your leadership strengths and look for learning opportunities to develop these strengths instead of always looking at your leadership gaps and trying to fix what does not come naturally to you.
- Assess your EI and SI and take action steps to improve both. EI and SI give you the opportunity to have greater impact and more success in your life and work.
- Take care of yourself by taking time away from work. Develop a mindfulness practice. Over time, this practice will help you be more present and calmer in your role as leader.

Supplemental Resources

- Tara Brach's website (www.tarabrach.com/): For mindfulness and other resources on self-compassion.
- Strengths-Based Leadership (www.gallup.com/cliftonstrengths/en/252137/home .aspx): For more information on developing your leadership strengths.
- Brené Brown's website (https://brenebrown.com/): For more information on leading and vulnerability.
- The Leadership Challenge (www.leadershipchallenge.com/): For more information on exemplary practices of leadership.
- Co-Active Institute (https://coactive.com/): For additional coaching and leadership development resources.

REFERENCES

1. Senge, P. *The Fifth Discipline: The Art & Practice of the Learning Organization.* Currency Doubleday; 2006.
2. Flores A, Risley K, Zanoni J, et al. Factors of success for transitioning from a scientific role to a supervisory leadership role in a federal public health agency. *Public Health Rep.* 2019; 134(5):466–471. doi:10.1177/0033354919867728.
3. Centers for Disease Control and Prevention. *10 Essential Public Health Services.* https:// www.cdc.gov/publichealthgateway/publichealthservices/essentialhealthservices.html. Updated March 18, 2021. Accessed March 28, 2021.

4. Kegan R, Laskow Lahey L. *Immunity to Change: How to Uncover It and Unlock Potential in Yourself and Your Organization.* Harvard Business School Publishing Corporation; 2009.

5. Goleman D, Boyatzis R, McKee A. *Primal Leadership: Unleashing the Power of Emotional Intelligence.* Harvard Business Review Press; 2013.

6. Kania J, Kramer M, Senge P. *The Water of Systems Change: Six Conditions of Systems Change.* https://www.fsg.org/publications/water_of_systems_change. Published May 2018. Accessed March 28, 2021.

7. David R. Relationships key to staying relevant amidst change. International City/County Management Association. https://icma.org/articles/relationships-key-staying-relevant-amidst-change. Accessed March 29, 2021.

8. DeSalvo KB, Wang YC, Harris A, Auerbach J, Koo D, O'Carroll P. Public Health 3.0: a call to action for public health to meet the challenges of the 21st century. *Prev Chronic Dis.* 2017;14:170017. doi:10.5888/pcd14.170017.

9. About John Snow. *The John Snow Archive and Research Companion.* https://johnsnow.matrix.msu.edu/aboutjohn.php. Accessed March 30, 2021.

10. Lillian Wald. *Henry Street Settlement.* https://www.henrystreet.org/about/our-history/lillian-wald/. Accessed March 30, 2021.

11. *Public Health Accreditation Board. Standards and Measures: Version 1.5.* https://www.phaboard.org/wp-content/uploads/PHABSM_WEB_LR1.pdf. Published December 2013. Accessed March 28, 2021.

12. Health Resources and Services Administration. *Maternal and Child Health Leadership Competencies. Version 4.0.* https://mchb.hrsa.gov/training/leadership-00.asp. Accessed March 28, 2021.

13. Maslow A. *The Psychology of Science: A Reconnaissance.* Harper & Row; 1966.

14. Leider J, Harper E, Bhartihapudi K, Castrucci B. Educational attainment of the public health workforce and its implications for workforce development. *J Public Health Manag Pract.* 2015;21(Suppl 6):s56–s68.

15. Koh H, Jacobson M. Fostering public health leadership. *J Public Health.* 2009;31(2):199–201.

16. Kouzes J, Posner B. *The Leadership Challenge: How to Make Extraordinary Things Happen in Organizations.* John Wiley & Sons, Inc.; 2017.

17. Whitworth L, Kimsey-House K, Kimsey-House H, Sandahl P. *Co-Active Coaching: New Skills for Coaching People Toward Success in Work and Life.* 2nd ed. Davies-Black; 2009.

18. Boyatzis R, McKee A. *Resonant Leadership.* Harvard Business School Publishing; 2005.

19. Rath T, Conchie B. *Strengths-Based Leadership: Great Leaders, Teams, and Why People Follow.* Gallup Press; 2008.

20. Bradberry T, Greaves J. *Emotional Intelligence 2.0.* TalentSmart; 2009.

21. Kabat Zinn J. *Defining Mindfulness.* Mindful website. https://www.mindful.org/jon-kabat-zinn-defining-mindfulness/. Published January 11, 2017. Accessed March 28, 2021.

22. Brach T. *How to Meditate.* https://www.tarabrach.com/howtomeditate/. Accessed March 28, 2021.

23. Magee R. *The Inner Work of Racial Justice: Healing Ourselves and Transforming Our Communities Through Mindfulness.* Penguin Random House; 2019.

5

Interpersonal Leadership: Effective Approaches for Systems Change

Patricia Moten Marshall, Christina R. Welter, and Samantha Cinnick

CHAPTER OBJECTIVES

As a result of this chapter, the practitioner will be able to:

- Describe a process that builds meaningful interpersonal connections for systems change.
- Name effective skills and techniques for building interpersonal leadership for systems change.
- Cite examples of application in practice.

INTRODUCTION

This chapter provides an overview of **Creative Interchange**, a behavioral science process that leaders can use to effect systems change at the interpersonal level.

THE IMPORTANCE OF INTERPERSONAL LEADERSHIP TO SYSTEMS CHANGE

Interpersonal leadership puts one's personal values, vision, and awareness of strengths into practice to develop effective relationships with others. This is vital for systems change because most public health system challenges are complex and there are often multiple perspectives regarding which root causes are accurate or the one to address first. Differing perspectives about these can result in a high degree of conflict about how to proceed or symptomatic fixes to individual pieces of the problem rather than the whole. Our ability to move forward to address these challenges in part stems from our ability to apply interpersonal leadership processes and skills to create authentic, meaningful relationships where diverse perspectives can be shared, understood, and explored synergistically to co-create generative visions of the future.[1]

Exercising interpersonal leadership requires being open to diverse perspectives while acknowledging one's personal worldviews and social identities, non judgmental listening and curiosity, and finding connections between seemingly unrelated situations. With this approach and set of skills, interpersonal leadership can serve as a powerful foundation to transformative, relational, and systems change. Interpersonal leadership can facilitate a shift in mental models about how to interact with others, helping to work toward jointly developed solutions that benefit the health of the whole and may not be evident to any of us individually. By deepening the quality of interpersonal connections and improving communication among actors in a system, especially among those with differing histories and viewpoints, we open new pathways and innovations to change the system for the better.

There are different approaches to fostering interpersonal leadership. For example, Goleman, Boyatzis, and McKee (2013) suggest that building social awareness (i.e., building empathy, organizational awareness, and service) and managing relationships (i.e., our ability to inspire, influence, manage conflict and work as a team, develop others, and serve as a catalyst for change) are two critical aspects of developing interpersonal strengths.[2] Our framework provides a holistic, profound, and innate approach to undertaking interpersonal leadership. **Creative Interchange** is both a philosophy and four-fold process that weaves in tangible skills that practitioners can use to unpack and build interpersonal systems change leadership strengths. This chapter focuses on describing **Creative Interchange** with tools and tips for implementation and illustrative practice-based examples.

CHALLENGES OF INTERPERSONAL INTERACTIONS

In the pursuit to address systems change through profound and effective relationships, challenges can occur that keep people from reaching their optimal potential and outcomes. As we speak with different people, diversity naturally surfaces in conversation. Diversity is when there is a perspective different than our own and it surfaces no matter whom you bring together. Humans are not clones. Each person brings to an interpersonal interaction their unique perspectives built on their origins, history, culture, and narratives. It is what we do with diversity when it surfaces that is important when leading systems change.

Let's explore what frequently happens when diversity surfaces. Initially, participants start discussing their own points of view. Focused on getting their point across, this can result in a volley of ideas without listening to the content or emotions behind all the perspectives presented. Each participant, invested in their own way of thinking, starts debating which idea is best. Often the goal is for the participants to convince others of the "correctness" of their approach and the "wrongness" of any others. Frequently, the debate turns into a division among the participants. The divergence generates an either/or situation around the topic, further polarizing participants. This polarization leads to four outcomes: divorce, agree to disagree, compromise, and groupthink (Exhibit 5.1).

CREATIVE INTERCHANGE AS A PROCESS FOR FACILITATING INTERPERSONAL INTERACTIONS

When it comes to interpersonal leadership, we must ask ourselves, "How do we solve the problem of polarity in order to achieve the level of thinking and interaction to accomplish complex systems change?" Leaders need a process to overcome unproductive debate, division, and polarization in interpersonal interaction to fully utilize diverse thoughts and perspectives. One way to do this is through the enabling process of **Creative Interchange**.

Creative Interchange, coined by Henry Nelson Wieman and further explored by his student Charles Palmgren, is the process, unique to human beings, through which we learn, change, and perform to our highest potential (Exhibit 5.2).

Although this chapter focuses on **Creative Interchange** at the individual and interpersonal level, it can also be applied to team and community leadership. One of the fundamental tenets of **Creative Interchange** is the belief that all people have intrinsic worth. To say this in a different way, no matter with whom you are interacting, their perspectives, insights, and ideas have value, and there is something that can be learned, appreciated, and gained from the interaction. Starting with this belief, leaders engage in the **Creative Interchange** process, which includes Authentic Interacting, Appreciative Understanding, Creative Integrating, and Expanding Capacity (see Figure 5.1).

EXHIBIT 5.1 Common Outcomes of Polarization

- Divorce: Participants remove themselves from the situation and decide not to continue interacting.
- Agree to disagree: Participants accept the situation and disengage in further discourse on the issue.
- Compromise: Both sides give up something for a less desirable outcome and everyone ends up losing.
- Groupthink: A participant may yield their idea because there is a louder, more popular, or more powerful voice that dominates and prevails, potentially reducing the final selected outcome's strength or innovative quality. May be the least optimal outcome of polarization.

EXHIBIT 5.2 Henry Nelson Wieman and Charles Palmgren Biographies

■ American philosopher and theologian Henry Nelson Wieman was born in 1884, the son of a Presbyterian minister in Richhill, Missouri. When he went to college, he intended to study journalism. One April evening in 1907, as he sat alone looking over the Missouri River in the faint light of dusk, a sudden conviction came over Wieman—a conviction that he should devote his life to *religious inquiry* and its central problem. The epiphany set the course for the rest of his life. He set out from that experience to discover what it is *that transforms the human mind* toward its *highest potential good*. He wanted to understand the experience that transforms human life and deserves one's ultimate commitment and highest devotion. He would eventually name the process **Creative Interchange**.

Less known to many of his biographers was his work in the final 10 years of his life (he died in 1975). In those closing years, he devoted his time to a deeper understanding of the psychological aspects of **Creative Interchange** and its value developing healthier families, groups, teams, and organizations. He, along with his student Dr. Charles Palmgren, were part of developing The Center for Creative Interchange in Des Moines, Iowa, in 1967.

■ Dr. Charles Palmgren's career spans roles as behavioral psychologist, therapist, international corporate consultant, and Episcopal priest. Inspired by his mentor, Palmgren has spent decades researching and writing about organizational development, human behavior, and human transformation. His undergraduate and master's degrees are in psychology and his PhD is in applied behavioral science and organizational development. Dr. Palmgren established SynerChange International in Atlanta, Georgia, and, with several affiliates, has sought to make **Creative Interchange** more accessible to individuals and organizations. He has authored two books that lend clarity to **Creative Interchange**—*The Chicken Conspiracy*[3] and *Ascent of the Eagle.*[4]

THE CREATIVE INTERCHANGE PROCESS

To learn, change, and perform to our highest potential within interpersonal interactions, leaders establish environments for the four components of **Creative Interchange**. Although, ideally, we would master each component before moving on to the next, a more appropriate metaphor for how a practitioner enters the **Creative Interchange** process might be an aerial view of a highway with four cloverleaf ramps leading into it. The process can occur in any sequence and anything can happen in an interpersonal interaction that can lead to a different place in the process. In this section of the chapter, each component will be introduced with a definition, the three conditions needed

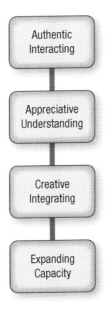

Figure 5.1 Creative Interchange process.

to achieve that component, and the skills and the techniques to master the component provided within the context of a real-world example.

Authentic Interacting

Authentic Interacting is the willingness and ability to bring one's genuine self, inclusive of stories, experiences, knowledge, skills, and preferences, to an interpersonal interaction. To authentically interact is to communicate what is on one's mind and share without pretense with one another; it requires leaders to be vulnerable and share what is unique and novel about themselves and their ideas while allowing others to do the same. What is key to supporting these behaviors is recognizing the courage it takes to show diversity of thought.

Engaging in Authentic Interacting involves two simultaneous behaviors. First, a person must be willing to share their self and ideas with integrity—to inform. If participants are truly sharing with integrity, every thought relevant to the topic of conversation is revealed. Second, a person must be willing to listen with humility—to learn. If participants are truly listening to learn, there is an emergence in the mind of something that was not there before, and each participant discovers a fresh perspective after the interaction. Such an interaction begins with a topic for discussion, without preconceived notions about what will materialize from the conversation. Ultimately, Authentic Interacting opens up the possibility for new perspectives shared, new ideas and connections generated, and innovations created toward systems change.

Creative Communication Versus Other Kinds of Communication

Wieman distinguishes communication that leads to **Creative Interchange** from other types of communication that we frequently encounter in our interpersonal leadership, such as deceptive, manipulative, reiterative, "muddleheaded," or "other directed person" communication (Exhibit 5.3).[5]

To encourage creative communication, leaders might ask themselves, "Am I doing anything in my leadership practice that is causing people to mask their true selves? What is keeping those around me from authentically interacting?" Removing those barriers will assist in facilitating creative communication and engaging in Authentic Interacting.

Three Conditions of Authentic Interacting

Three conditions encourage an environment for Authentic Interacting. The first condition is psychological safety. Psychological safety refers to an individual's perception that there will not be negative consequences for taking an interpersonal risk, such as asking questions, offering new ideas, or admitting a mistake. A person who perceives high psychological safety feels confident that they will not be punished or embarrassed for raising a concern or innovative approach.[6] The second condition is trust. Relationships built on trust encourage vulnerability because there is an understanding that sensitive information will not be used against them. The last condition is an openness to others' perspectives. To allow room for new ideas to emerge, the mind must be open to all other possibilities and not restricted to current ways of thinking. When these three conditions

---

EXHIBIT 5.3 Definitions of Communication Types

- Creative communication: Communication leading to an emergence in the mind of something that wasn't there before
- Deceptive communication: Concealing what we do not want others to recognize
- Manipulative communication: Attempting to suppress the thoughts and feelings of others insofar as they run counter to what one wants to communicate
- Reiterative communication: Repetitious and no new information
- "Muddleheaded" communication: Communicating odds and ends, but there is no information to integrate
- "Other directed person" communication: Putting on a false front or communicating differently based on the audience or situation to please others; this might be the most frequent kind of communication seen in organizations today

Source: Wieman HN. *Man's Ultimate Commitment.* Southern Illinois University Press; 1958.

are met, it clears the ways for people to communicate with directness, low distortion, and high congruence; actively listen to both facts and feelings expressed by others; and communicate in a manner that generates trust and credibility with each other.

Authentic Interacting in Practice

Systems change leaders are no strangers to resistance. Resistance is defined as the "physiological and psychological responses to change that manifest in specific behaviors." It might look like disengagement; reduced productivity; conflict; negativity; avoidance; building barriers; or emotional expressions of fear, sadness, and anxiety.[7] Significant change is always accompanied by resistance; it is human nature. As resistance appears, it is important to uncover the reason for and accelerant of the resistance to minimize it. When the actors in the system express resistance overtly instead of covertly, it can help their stakeholders relent and accept, or even embrace, the change. To open dialogue about resistance to change, leaders can ensure that an environment exists for Authentic Interacting. Let's look at an example.

Carol, a new leader, is in the process of making changes at her organization. She is intent on hearing the senior team's thoughts about the changes and has found them reluctant to share any concerns. Carol hires a consultant to interview the senior team members and it is apparent that no one thinks Carol is open to hearing what they have to say. They cite the resignation of a team member who had spoken up about their concerns as a sign that they, too, might be taking an interpersonal risk if they speak out. What might Carol do to establish an environment for the senior team to be authentic and share their concerns about the change?

Authentic Interacting Skills and Techniques: Exercises for Practitioners

There are several skills and techniques Carol could choose from to engage in Authentic Interacting with her senior team, including balancing advocacy and inquiry, communicating to all styles, and listening with all senses.

Balancing Advocacy and Inquiry: This approach is about spending the same amount of time sharing your best knowledge as you do asking about other's best knowledge. Balancing advocacy and inquiry might look like providing your best thinking and allotting the same amount of time and energy to listening to another's perspectives and ideas. For example, you might limit the sharing of your perspective to 45-second soundbites, and then pause and ask for insights from the other person.

Communicating to All Styles: Every person has a communication preference; some people like to talk about the big picture while others like to talk about granularities, some people like to talk about ideas while other people like to talk about events, and some people like to talk about the future while others like to talk about the past. These are only a few examples of the breadth of communication preferences you might see in your interpersonal interactions. If you are not aware of or open to listening to different communication styles, you may miss opportunities for Authentic Interacting. When engaging in Authentic Interacting, you should show an appreciation for how others communicate and seek to match your communication to their style preferences.

There is an easy to administer "Communicating Styles Survey" tool that can be used to gain insight into your communication style preference and preferences of others. The "Starter Kit" provides information about how to use the results of the survey (see Supplemental Resources list).

   Listening With Our Senses: Listening is so much more than the words and syntax used in our messages. To accurately interpret what other people are trying to say and for other people to accurately interpret what you are trying to say, you should strive to use as many senses as possible to absorb the information and allow others to use their senses as well. When listening or speaking, pay equal or more attention to nonverbal cues (Exhibit 5.4).

Applying Authentic Interacting Skills and Techniques

Now that Carol is equipped with these three skills and techniques, she can take a different approach with the senior team. Originally, Carol would spend a large amount of time in meetings advocating for her ideas, moving on quickly after asking for any questions or concerns from others, and requesting team members to send any concerns to her by email. Additionally, Carol was a naturally optimistic person who preferred to talk about the "big picture" while some wanted more details about how the change would affect individual people and were nervous that Carol would reject any comments she perceived as cynical. She also met with the senior staff members across from a huge, intimidating desk that represented a power dynamic. After learning about some of the barriers to Authentic Interacting. Carol spent less time speaking about her points of view and more time asking about and listening to the team's ideas and concerns. She considered the communication styles of her team members and chose her words more

EXHIBIT 5.4 Authentic Interacting Skill—Listening With All Senses

* 7% Verbal Listening

   * Words
   * Syntax

* 38% Nonverbal Listening

   * Volume (loud/soft)
   * Pitch (high/low)
   * Rate (fast/slow)
   * Pauses (many/few, long/short)

* 55% Nonvocal Seeing

   * Facial expressions
   * Body posture
   * Gestures (e.g., fingers, hands, arms, and legs)

Source: Mehrabian A, Wiener M. Decoding of inconsistent communications. *Journal of Personality and Social Psychology.* 1967;6(1):109–114. doi:10.1037/h0024532.

carefully when responding to concerns about the change. She provided more details about the change to facilitate a more robust conversation about resistance. Finally, she used one-on-one meetings with team members to obtain their concerns, in person, and met with team members at a round table that gave the perception of shared power.

Appreciative Understanding

Appreciative Understanding is welcoming diversity that has surfaced, seeking to understand why this person thinks differently, and valuing what others understand and value. Through Appreciative Understanding, leaders affirm that others' contributions are important and acknowledge that the group's achievements are attributable to every team member's input.

Three Conditions of Appreciative Understanding

In this component of **Creative Interchange**, three important conditions are curiosity, capacity for ambiguity, and the ability to "hold reality lightly." To appreciatively understand, leaders need curiosity or a sincere desire to learn why someone thinks differently than they do and where that different perspective originates. Second, leaders tolerate ambiguity and feel comfortable not having all the answers. By sitting with ambiguity, leaders leave room to seek many different viewpoints instead of jumping to solutions. Finally, leaders acknowledge that their perspective does not represent reality any more than another's perspective—that is, the leader's way is not the only way. Realizing that reality is created by our sensory experience makes it a little easier to lay down our current reality and embrace new perspectives.

When these conditions are met, there will be a willingness and ability to create an open climate where differences can be surfaced; delay forming negative judgments about others' ideas, beliefs, feelings, attitudes, behavior, or concerns; empathize with others and view their perspective as legitimate for them; and value diversity and identify positive characteristics about other viewpoints.

Appreciative Understanding in Practice

To recognize Appreciative Understanding in practice, let's look at an example. Jeffrey is currently working at an organization that has made a commitment to advancing diversity, equity, and inclusion (DEI). However, despite this promise by both the organization and Jeffrey, the organization has been having a hard time keeping a DEI director in the position for more than 1 year. Jeffrey hires a consultant to interview the past two incumbents to understand their motivations for leaving. Both people say that Jeffrey was using the DEI director role for show and was not serious about DEI work. Although Jeffrey would tell them he wanted change, his actions did not match his words. As an example, both DEI directors reported that when they would give him recommendations to reach the organization's DEI goals, implementing those recommendations depended on if Jeffrey already expected their proposals. If Jeffrey had been expecting something else, then he would say the organization was not ready. Without appreciating the innovative recommendations of future DEI directors, the interviewees were afraid that no one would be able to stay for more than a year in the position. What might Jeffrey do to remain curious and see the value in approaches presented by a new DEI director?

Appreciative Understanding Skills and Techniques: Exercises for Practitioners

Some of the skills and techniques Jeffrey could use to practice Appreciative Understanding include confirmed paraphrasing, empathetic or empathic listening, and finding positives and drawbacks.

Confirmed Paraphrasing: Confirmed paraphrasing is a way to ensure the interpretation of the listener is equal to the intention of the speaker. There are three levels to confirmed paraphrasing—content, affect, and valuative. At the content level, you can confirm the intention of the speaker by feeding back the speaker's message in your own words. At the affect level, you can verify that you understood the underlying emotions of the message and that the interpreted emotions matched the speaker's intention. As a listener, you can check emotional intention by offering statements to confirm their emotional state, such as "It seems like this topic makes you really angry." At the valuative level, you are paraphrasing what is most important to the speaker—that is, the core of the message or what the speaker values. Perhaps a speaker is explaining how important it is to find a job that offers a flexible work schedule, work from home options, and regular review of the workload by the manager. As a savvy listener, you might infer that the speaker values work–life balance and would want to confirm that by offering the statement, "So, it sounds like work–life balance is really important to you." You should assure that the speaker agrees with your paraphrasing before moving on; if the speaker says that the paraphrase didn't match their intention, you would seek to clarify further.

Empathetic or Empathic Listening: If you are seeking to understand appreciatively, you should be attuned to your level of listening (Exhibit 5.5).

Although listening at the attentive or active level gives more time and attention to the speaker's content, it falls short of listening to what the speaker means. To truly practice Appreciative Understanding, the most impactful listening is empathetic or empathic because this type of listening requires you to stop listening from your point of view and value system and to find meaning from the speaker's point of view and value system. This type of listening is a difficult skill to learn; however, practicing valuative level paraphrasing, expressing a time when you had a similar experience or feeling to the speaker, and compassionate expression (i.e., helping the speaker solve their problem or handle the situation) can help increase your ability to listen empathetically or empathically.

Finding Positives and Drawbacks: This is a practice to find value in all perspectives offered. This technique involves extracting both the positive elements and drawbacks from the contributions made by yourself and by others. Illuminating positives and drawbacks demonstrates a willingness to assess and appreciate all viewpoints. For example, when you are meeting with another person and each of you have different suggestions for a solution, you might pull out a piece of paper, draw a line down the

EXHIBIT 5.5 Five Levels of Listening

- Ignoring or passive: The listener is not giving any attention to what the speaker is saying.
- Pretend: The listener gives the impression that they are listening (e.g., nodding at the speaker's words), but they are not giving the speaker their full attention.
- Selective: The listener hears some things and not others, often listening when the message feels relevant to them or contains the message they want.
- Attentive or active: The listener gives the speaker their time and attention but is short of empathetic or empathic listening because they are still listening from their own frame of reference.
- Empathetic or empathic: The listener pays attention to the speaker's body language, intonation, and content to gain an overall collective appreciation of how the other person is feeling. The listener is putting themselves inside the other person's frame of reference.

Source: Covey SR. *The 7 Habits of Highly Effective People: Powerful Lessons in Personal Change.* 25th anniversary ed. Simon & Schuster; 2004.

center, and the two of you highlight the positives in column 1 and drawbacks in column 2 for each solution. It is amazing how illuminating this exercise can be toward finding the optimal solution.

Applying Appreciative Understanding Skills and Techniques

Jeffrey applied the skills and techniques for Appreciative Understanding with the next DEI director hired, Michala. From the beginning, Jeffrey stressed the importance of authenticity in the interactions between himself and Michala. He confessed to her what he had learned from the interviews with the previous DEI directors and committed himself to doing better. During their conversations, he used confirmed paraphrasing to ensure his understanding of her intent. He asked her to do the same. He sought to put himself in her shoes as she explained her motivations and challenges. When she offered a new proposal for moving toward the goals established, they would take the time to delineate both the positives and drawbacks. Most notably, when he disagreed with her way of thinking or ideas, he would listen most ardently, paraphrase at the affect and valuative levels, and illuminate the positives. He and Michala initiated a practice in which the person on the receiving end of a new idea or solution first identified the positives of a new idea or solution and the contributor then identified the drawbacks. Michala acknowledged that even though all her proposals were not accepted, she felt that consideration was always given to them. She stated that when a proposal did not move forward, it was typically a joint decision between herself and Jeffrey. Jeffrey acknowledged that taking the extra time to vet the proposals helped him confront his own biases, get out of his comfort zone, and implement some innovative new programs in the organization.

Creative Integrating

Creative Integrating may be the most difficult component and is defined as letting go of polarizing viewpoints and instead embracing complexity and paradox to find the connections between alleged contradictions. There is an emphasis on using "right-brain thinking" or imagination, creativity, and intuition to create something new and different. During Creative Integrating, participants are actively seeking to combine outcomes that are inclusive of the strengths of ideas, emotions, and values surfaced in the first two phases. Creative Integrating generates results that are more than and different from what one could achieve in isolation.

Three Conditions of Creative Integrating

Conditions to engage in Creative Integrating include connecting, imagining, and playing. First, leaders create space for revealing connections between things that are connected in ways that are not readily apparent and help others find those connections. Second, leaders establish environments where people can tap into their "right-brain thinking" and unearth and create ideas, images, or concepts. Lastly, Creative Integrating at times benefits from removing oneself from the serious, practical, or purposeful to engage in activities that increase one's propensity to dream, visualize possibilities, and notice unexpected connections. Leaders can do this by encouraging those they work with to recognize fun and play as pathways to creativity and releasing the restrictions of our linear thinking. If these conditions are met, an ability and willingness to tolerate ambiguity; be persistent in the struggle for new possibilities; and modify one's own views, beliefs, and behaviors are unleashed. Additionally, participants can generate creative ways of merging diverse perspectives into new, mutually supported alternatives as well as identify issues, concepts, and situations that cannot or should not be integrated.

Creative Integrating in Practice

An example of Creative Integrating can be seen through the story of Sophia and Immanuel. Sophia and Immanuel are senior leaders and peers at an organization working on a significant change initiative. Both Sophia and Immanuel have different opinions about the next steps for the project and both are sure that their approach is the right one. Sophia and Immanuel consult their supervisor and explain the situation. The supervisor acknowledges their dilemma and says if Sophia and Immanuel can't find a solution together, she will intervene. Sophia and Immanuel want to show their supervisor that they can work together without succumbing to groupthink or compromise to move the change initiative forward. What might Sophia and Immanuel do to combine the best of both of their ideas to create something amazing?

Creative Integrating Skills and Techniques: Exercises for Practitioners

The skills and techniques Sophia and Immanuel might use to creatively integrate their ideas are plentiful. In this section, we highlight five exercises practitioners can use to facilitate this component.

Yes, And: One simple way to build your receptivity to creative thinking is to re-move "yes, but" from your vocabulary and insert "yes, and" instead. By using "yes, and" you provide an environment to develop creative ideas rather than start with critiques that lead ideas to wither. For example, when someone offers an idea, you can answer with an enthusiastic "yes, and" and use this phrase to build upon the idea.

Three Plusses and a Wish: Another powerful way to build creative ideas is the technique "Three Plusses and a Wish." This approach is helpful for finding value and continuing to encourage an idea you disagree with—in fact, it may reduce the tension felt between two parties that are debating ideas they feel strongly about. To practice this approach, when an idea is presented, first find three things that are positive about the idea. Then, turn the negative aspects of the idea into a wish statement (i.e., what you wish was different about the idea that would make it more amenable). Now, a new idea that builds on the positive and responds to the wish can be offered until a resolution can be endorsed by all parties. In addition to supporting the person who offered the idea, engaging in "Three Plusses and a Wish" recognizes that ideas are made of discrete pieces that can be rearranged, combined, and improved as opposed to concepts for which you must challenge their legitimacy (Table 5.1).

Finding Connections: A third skill is being able to find connections between seemingly unconnected things. To practice this, select two objects and brainstorm all possible connections. For example, you could ask yourself, "What is the connection between the moon and floor? What is the connection between infectious disease and a textbook?" These questions may seem silly; however, this quick exercise repeated on a regular basis forces your brain to stop "either/or" thinking and embrace "both/and" thinking.

TABLE 5.1 Example of Three Plusses and a Wish Technique

HOW TO DO IT	EXAMPLE	
	IDEA	TECHNIQUE
When you encounter a perspective or idea that you disagree with: ■ Find three positive aspects of the idea that you sincerely believe are relevant	I think the meeting should be extended to 4 hours.	Extending the meeting to 4 hours has several positive benefits: ■ It will ensure we touch upon all the issues on the table ■ It will give us the time to hear all the varied perspectives on the most salient issues ■ It will increase the likelihood that we can submit the proposal on time
■ Share what you do not like or disagree with using a "wish" statement		My wish is that 4 hours will not cause participants to find an excuse to leave the meeting early or not attend at all, as there are so many pressing priorities with which people are faced.

Analogies and Metaphors: A fourth technique to heighten "right-brain thinking" is using analogies and metaphors. Both are powerful tools to help look at things in new ways. You can use them to conjure up images in the mind that otherwise would not be there. One example of an analogy might be, "This conversation we're having is like a child trying to convince their grandmother that their parents would let them eat as many cookies as they want." An example of a metaphor might be, "This is the Super Bowl of grants that we are writing." Try using an analogy or metaphor when you want to ensure the other person appreciates the point you are trying to make or to link what you're saying to something with which the other person might be more familiar.

Reframing: Lastly, to engage in Creative Integrating, you might become skilled in reframing. Reframing is the process of identifying and then changing the way events, concepts, situations, perspectives and emotions are viewed in order to generate new possibilities. There are different ways to reframe. One might be to take something perceived as negative and turn it into a positive. An example might be one person commenting, "Our turnover rate is horrible, and I don't see how it's going to change, the way this organization is heading." You might reframe this comment by saying, "These openings from turnover give us an opportunity to hire individuals for which the job is truly a great fit." When problem-solving, you might reframe by moving the challenge from today to the future (e.g., "How might we look at this problem if we were 10 years into the future and everything is digitized?"). There are many exercises to practice reframing, with the goal of changing how you see the problem to imagine the possibilities (see Supplemental Resources for more exercises).

Applying Creative Integrating Skills and Techniques

Sophia and Immanuel were introduced to **Creative Interchange** at a workshop they attended together on leading change and are now equipped with new skills and techniques for Creative Integrating. As a first step, they decided to add levity to their meetings on the project. Each meeting began with the exercising of their right brains, like a warm-up activity one might do when arriving at the gym. The activity was to find six connections assigned by the other person (e.g., What is the connection between this pencil and our senior leadership team? What is the connection between your eyeglasses and this project? What is the connection between cheese and our supervisor?).

Additionally, Sophia and Immanuel agreed that whenever either of them uttered the word "but" without replacing it with the word "and," that person had to take a quick hike around whichever room they were in (it took about a month for the word "but" to be erased from their deliberations). They also committed to using the "Three Plusses and a Wish" technique for reactions to ideas, suggestions, or approaches that initially were met with negativity. Intriguingly, most of the time they could not remember the initial objection after completing the three positives and often came up with a better solution after building on the plusses and addressing the wishes.

When it came to facilitating play, Sophia and Immanuel were made aware of business board games designed to support the implementation of change initiatives. They purchased one and were impressed by how playing a game surfaced consideration for merging their respective approaches. On occasion, when the conference room in which they met wasn't yielding any new insights, Sophia and Immanuel would move their meeting outside or to a coffee shop down the street. On days they worked remotely from each other, they would take a break whenever they felt stuck and reconvene after a 5-minute rejuvenation period. They agreed the rejuvenation period could not be used to perform other work. Sophia and Immanuel, and their supervisor, were struck by how Creative Integrating allowed them to come back to their supervisor with a collaboratively endorsed approach and strengthen their relationship to the point where they now truly enjoyed working together.

Expanding Capacity

When Expanding Capacity, leaders act upon what has emerged and commit to continually learning and improving upon it. Expanding Capacity is a two-fold commitment in which leaders promise to act now on what they have, knowing it is not perfect, and continually strive to transform to the best they now know. In the process of **Creative Interchange**, there is a realization that you never arrive at the optimal outcome, that there is always more to be learned and achieved. The capacity to grow from continual engagement in **Creative Interchange** is limitless. At some point, though, action is needed to take advantage of the current thinking, benefit from the change that occurs and progress made, and then receive feedback from those actions and initiate the next improvement process.

Three Conditions of Expanding Capacity

Three conditions for Expanding Capacity are discipline, skilled action, and commitment. To enable change, there needs to be a disciplined and systematic approach, such as an implementation plan and careful consideration of how to move forward. Those who take action must be skilled. Attention should be given to whom the assignment is given to coordinate implementation. Who performs key roles during change and their level of preparedness to effectively perform the role are paramount to whether change is successful. To this end, the commitment of individuals and groups who can sponsor the change is one of the most significant determinants to enabling change.

If the conditions are met for this phase of **Creative Interchange**, there will be an ability and willingness in our interpersonal interactions to establish overall strategies and specific measurable goals and objectives, to monitor progress and supply the necessary reinforcement to ensure success. It also includes implementation at a speed and in a manner that acknowledges the needs of individuals and recognition that plans may need to be modified to bring relevance to the current reality.

Expanding Capacity in Practice

Two CEOs from separate organizations were pleased with the outcome of their deliberations. There was sizable grant funding available if they could respond to the request for proposal with a collaborative effort and a "bold solution." They had come up with something that neither of them had anticipated when they began their negotiations. Early in their discussions they had decided not to compromise and to remain in discussion until both felt they had a resolution that would be a win–win for each of their organizations and the constituents they serve, and they had succeeded. They recognized that the resolution was not perfect, and they knew that they must act now to seize the opportunity and could improve the idea over time. How do the CEOs and their respective organizations move forward and expand the capacity of their organizations with this grant funding?

Expanding Capacity Skills and Techniques: Exercises for Practitioners

Four skills and techniques the two CEOs might choose for Expanding Capacity are illuminated here, including implementation planning, adopting a growth mindset, action learning, and celebration.

Implementation Planning: It takes tenacity to move from where you are today to a new desired state. An implementation plan helps you think through the various strategies and tactics to take during change and the resources needed. Plans articulate the goals or vision to be achieved so you can, as the saying goes, "keep your attention on your intention." Individuals or groups performing key roles are delineated, with consideration given to skill-building needs. Communication is mapped out. Milestones are highlighted. Plans are also refined as the landscape changes and new approaches become necessary. As a public health professional, you may already use several frameworks for implementation planning; you can continue to use these processes and customize them to include systems thinking considerations. Also, there is a business board game called "ChangeABLE—A Workshop in a Box" that addresses many considerations for implementation planning (see Supplemental Resources list).

Adopt a "Growth Mindset": To get new results, you must be open to learning and trying new things in order to grow as practitioners and leaders. Expanding Capacity benefits from leaders seeking to learn more, develop new habits, and practice new skills. The book *Mindset: The New Psychology of Success* provides useful insights into adopting a "growth mindset," which is the belief that your "most basic abilities can be developed through dedication and hard work—brains and talent are just the starting point."[8] The book posits that a love of learning and resilience is essential for great accomplishment.[8]

Action Learning: Action learning is a capacity-building process and leadership tool that fosters interpersonal dialogue and systems thinking to help practitioners solve problems in their own organizations and communities. As opposed to quality improvement, which usually focuses on a particular program or task, action learning explores a complex problem in practice through a process of shared learning and action. Led by a coach facilitator who promotes critical thinking and inquiry, a group works collaboratively to develop a shared definition of a complex problem, develop and explore critical questions about this problem, collect new information and gain new skills to address the problem, and work to identify collective action.[9] To integrate action learning into your practice, you might enlist the help of a World Institute of Action Learning (WIAL) certified coach to take your group through the process (see the Supplemental Resources list for more information on WIAL).

Celebrate: Knowing your work is never done makes it imperative that you acknowledge key milestones and successes for the actions taken thus far. Celebration invigorates the weary, appreciates the efforts, and encourages forward movement. For example, throughout the month, take time to note small wins by your team. Ask your team to regularly take screenshots of emails with positive feedback and share articles where their work was recognized or keep written notes of their daily or weekly accomplishments. At the end of the month, compile the stories of success and share them with the whole team. This can even be done collaboratively.

Applying Expanding Capacity Skills and Techniques

The two CEOs establish the conditions for the successful implementation of their newly funded initiative. Each CEO selects one of the senior leaders from their respective organizations to lead a joint task force to oversee implementation. They ensure the leaders are skilled in moving initiatives like this forward. An implementation plan is developed that will guide the initiative. The CEOs recognize their role to be out front and communicating the importance of this initiative and their commitment to its success, sending encouraging messages, ensuring the resources are in place, monitoring progress, and sustaining their support throughout. At the same time, the CEOs remain committed to gaining feedback and learning how to improve what has been put in place.

CHAPTER SUMMARY

Interpersonal leadership for systems change is an ability to create, foster, and sustain meaningful, authentic relationships whereby diverse perspectives can be shared, appreciated, and applied to generate new visions of the future. Engaging in a **Creative Interchange** process gives leaders both a philosophy and guide to facilitate relationships that influence systems change in four important ways. First, Authentic Interacting seeks to create environments and connections in ways that build trust. This allows individuals to feel valued and heard and to become vulnerable enough to share their diverse perspectives. Second, Appreciative Understanding fosters an environment of listening and self-reflection whereby we truly want to listen and seek different viewpoints and pathways that help expand our view of the systems and paths forward. Third, Creative Integrating means we will find connections and synergies between ideas in different ways. This helps to foster innovation and new ideas rather than following the same path as before. Finally, Expanding Capacity encourages leaders to embrace their bold new thinking and take the first steps to implement while committing to continually revising and improving the change.

Often leaders might find themselves at different points in the **Creative Interchange** process. To quickly determine where you might be in your interpersonal leadership for any situation, use Table 5.2 to identify at which phase of the **Creative Interchange** process you might be arriving and recognize the tools to facilitate **Creative Interchange** at each phase.

Key Messages

- Addressing public health system challenges hinges on our ability to apply interpersonal leadership processes and skills to create authentic relationships where multiple, diverse perspectives about the root causes of the problem and ways to move forward can be shared, understood, and explored to create a future desired state.

TABLE 5.2 Creative Interchange Components, Conditions, and Skills/Techniques

PROCESS COMPONENT	CONDITIONS	SKILLS/TECHNIQUES
Authentic Interacting: The willingness and ability to bring one's genuine self, inclusive of stories, experiences, knowledge, skills, and preferences, to an interpersonal interaction.	Psychological safety Trust Openness	Balance advocacy and inquiry Communicating to all styles Listening with all senses
Appreciative Understanding: The ability to welcome the diversity that has been surfaced, seek to understand why this person thinks differently, and value what others understand and value.	Curiosity Capacity for ambiguity Hold reality lightly	Confirmed paraphrasing Empathetic or empathic listening Finding positives and drawbacks
Creative Integrating: Letting go of polarizing viewpoints and instead embracing complexity and paradox to find the connections between alleged contradictions.	Connecting Imagining Playing	"Yes, and" "Three plusses and a wish" Finding connections Analogies/metaphors Reframing
Expanding Capacity: Two-fold commitment where leaders promise to act now on what they have, knowing it is not perfect, and continually strive to transform the best they now know.	Discipline Skilled action Commitment	Implementation planning Adopt a "growth mindset" Action learning Celebrate

- Regardless of the idea being presented, every person's perspectives, insights, and ideas have value and there is something to be appreciated, learned, and gained from all interpersonal interactions.
- **Creative Interchange**, a process encompassing the four components of Authentic Interacting, Appreciative Understanding, Creative Integrating, and Expanding Capacity, is a useful framework for fully appreciating, learning from, and utilizing diverse thoughts and perspectives in systems change work.

Tips

- Prepare to implement **Creative Interchange** by encouraging the conditions necessary for Authentic Interacting, Appreciative Understanding, Creative Integrating, and Expanding Capacity. Evaluate the environment to see where conditions are already strong for **Creative Interchange** to take hold and where conditions need to be supported.

- Model the skills and techniques for the four components. For example, skills like "Yes, And" and "Three Plusses and a Wish" are powerful tools for building creative ideas, but they may seem awkward or unfamiliar to some. Systems change leaders should embrace these skills and perform them with enthusiasm to develop norms that incorporate the **Creative Interchange** process in their work.
- Keep in mind that the **Creative Interchange** process can happen in any sequence and that the nature of an interpersonal interaction can lead someone to start with any of the four components.

Supplemental Resources

- Identifying Communications Styles—Communications Styles Technology (materials that can be used to illuminate an individual's behavioral and communication style profile): https://cst-tap.com/about-us/
- Reframing Exercise—The Six Conversations (developed by Peter Block, these conversations provide a new way to talk and engage in community building): www.asmallgroup.net/pages/content/6_conversations.html
- How to Adopt a Growth Mindset—*Mindset: The New Psychology of Success: How We Can Learn to Fulfill Our Potential* by Carol Dweck: www.penguinrandomhouse.com/books/44330/mindset-by-carol-s-dweck-phd/
- World Institute for Action Learning—Information about action learning coaching and working with a certified coach: https://wial.org/
- ChangeABLE—A Workshop in a Box—a Tool for Leading Organizational & Professional Change board game—co-creators Patricia Moten Marshall and Barb McLennan: ChangeABLEgame.com

REFERENCES

1. Senge P, Hamilton H, Kania J. The dawn of system leadership. *Stanf Soc Innov Rev.* 2015;13(1):27–33. doi:10.48558/YTE7-XT62.
2. Goleman D, Boyatzis RE, McKee A. *Primal Leadership: Unleashing the Power of Emotional Intelligence.* Harvard Business Press; 2013.
3. Palmgren C, Hagen S. *Chicken Conspiracy: Breaking the Cycle of Personal Stress & Organizational Mediocrity.* Recovery Communications; 1999.
4. Palmgren C. *Ascent of the Eagle: Being and Becoming Your Best.* Innovative InterChange Press; 2008.
5. Wieman HN. *Man's Ultimate Commitment.* Southern Illinois University Press; 1958.
6. *Guide: Understand Team Effectiveness.* re:Work website. https://rework.withgoogle.com/guides/understanding-team-effectiveness/steps/introduction/. Published March 10, 2018. Accessed January 7, 2021.
7. Managing resistance to change overview. Prosci website. https://www.prosci.com/resources/articles/managing-resistance-to-change. Published October 1, 2020. Accessed January 7, 2021.
8. Dweck C. *Mindset: The New Psychology of Success: How We Can Learn to Fulfill Our Potential.* Ballantine Book; 2008.
9. Marquardt MJ, Leonard HS, Freedman AM, Hill CC. *Action Learning for Development Leaders and Organizations: Principles, Strategies, and Cases.* American Psychological Association; 2009.

6

Organizational Leadership: "We Are the Ones We Have Been Waiting For"*

Mary F. Morten and Geneva Porter

CHAPTER OBJECTIVES

By the end of this chapter, the practitioner will be able to:

- Describe a process to foster organizational change with a racial equity, access, diversity, and inclusion lens.
- Discuss the importance of a simultaneous power shift and dismantling of longstanding organizational practices and policies to elevate the voices of those who are most often ignored, undervalued, or silenced.
- Apply leadership strategies to address systems change aligning with a public health perspective grounded in community building and collaboration.

INTRODUCTION

With the broadest of endeavors to improve community health, the elimination of health disparities is tantamount to addressing the social determinants of health as the sector has come to understand racism as a public health issue.[2] True systems change considers the intersectionality of its participants in a community health environment will be successful only with a direct and intentional inclusion of racial equity, access, diversity, and inclusion (READI).

Understanding the social determinants of health as the social conditions where people live, learn, play, and work impact a myriad of health and quality-of-life outcomes.

* The subtitle of this chapter is borrowed from June Jordan's "Poem for South African Women."[1]

Black, Indigenous, and People of Color (BIPOC) communities are disproportionately impacted by the inequities in systems that discriminate and exclude these historically marginalized voices. To address pervasive inequities in the community health system, a concerted and sustained effort toward the adoption of READI principles and actions is the primary and central opportunity for building equitable and healthy communities. The following scenario is an example of longstanding practices and policies within an organization's culture that can hinder this work.

> *A small liberal arts college in the Pacific Northwest has started working with a consulting group to deepen its efforts on diversity, equity, and inclusion. The college has been run for many years by the same group of administrators, with the majority of the team having been in various leadership roles for close to 20 years. As the trainings are completed, it becomes clear that at least two of the executive team members have concerns about the work and at least one person has made anti-Black statements—not with the consulting group itself—however, they are putting up roadblocks to what will be necessary to effectuate real change in the organization. The two executives have made several concerning statements that could potentially hinder any additional progress. As the READI work continues, constructive feedback on processes is met with resistance and defensiveness, and therefore who decides who will hold the power to make decisions does not change. The consultants are encouraged to move forward, yet they are expected to do so with minimal interaction with the executive team members who are the most resistant to the work.*

As a national consulting group that dedicates a major part of its practice to READI support, the preceding scenario is not an unusual dynamic. Internal team members who are necessary to carry out the critical work around READI in an organization cannot be "worked around" as it flies in the face of the very work that READI practices seek to uncover and dispel.

As illustrated in the scenario, unless there is a power shift in an organization, along with the dismantling of longstanding practices and policies that do not elevate the voices of those who are most often ignored, undervalued, or silenced, there will not be any substantial progress made on diversity, racial equity, and inclusion efforts, particularly within public health efforts.

Organizational leadership, loosely defined as a management approach to encourage staff to follow a clear, compelling, and strategic vision, is one capacity that *must* be achieved if there is to be any success in systems change in building equitable organizations and ultimately the work that practitioners do in our organizations and communities to improve community health. Leading with a commitment to consistent communication and respectful dialogue when differences occur while working toward collaboration is fundamental to lasting systems change. Systems leaders work across wildly divergent ideas and opinions and build coalitions toward mutual goals for change. Understanding the role of power and privilege in this work and being willing to disrupt processes that do not encourage full inclusion of all team members are critical steps toward building teams and accountability. This describes working toward a READI culture in an organization. The organizational leaders must motivate team members and secure buy-in and ownership for there to be significant and visible change. Successful organizational leadership also means that moving toward large-scale action requires an understanding of the collective impact in the sector. It means fighting against the default positions of individualism that are often organized around resistance toward innovation and the fundamental shift in what power and access look like in any system.

GETTING THERE FROM HERE: TENETS FOR BUILDING A READI CULTURE

As indicated in *Leading From the Emerging Future*, authors Otto Scharmer and Katrin Kaeufer[3] describe three "openings" that support the transformation of systems. These three openings support and collaborate with systems leaders who will ultimately make institutional change happen. The openings are: (a) how leaders must focus on the larger system; (b) how leaders must foster reflection and generate conversation; and (c) how leaders shift from reactive problem-solving to co-creating the future. All three of these tenets align with the steps necessary to build a READI culture. From a public health perspective, leaders of organizations within the public health system must go beyond their own silos in order to collectively work with those across the system. They then must shift from a mindset of focusing on individual organizational service delivery and programming to jointly envisioning a more READI state across the system. Systems leaders must prioritize the *bold vision,* the power to inspire, engage, and compel people to do better and work toward a common goal. The bold vision is mentioned often and is understood by all team members. From the moment anyone engages with an organization, they understand and become a part of the bold vision. It is baked into its internal operations and external engagement and is favored over a more traditional, less effective, and equity-absent approach.

DEFINING RACIAL EQUITY, ACCESS, DIVERSITY, AND INCLUSION

One of the first steps in building a READI culture is to address a foundational understanding of terms and concepts.

Racial equity is the condition that would be achieved if one's racial identity no longer predicted, in a statistical sense, how one fares. When using the term, practitioners should be thinking about equity as one part of justice, and thus also include work to address root causes of inequities, not just their manifestation. This includes elimination of policies, practices, attitudes, and cultural messages that reinforce differential outcomes by identities or fail to eliminate them. Given that race remains one of the primary indicators of one's success in this country, achieving racial equity means that race no longer dictates one's socioeconomic outcome.

Without racial equity, there will be no gender equity, LGBTQ equity, or disability equity, to name a few systems of oppression that intersect with race and must be addressed for any lasting systemic change.

Access is the intentional elimination of barriers and the cultivation of attitudes, behaviors, policies, procedures, and both physical and virtual spaces to create and provide inclusive opportunities for people of all abilities and experiences to meaningfully engage and contribute to and within physical and virtual places, including but not limited to personal and professional meetings and other events, conversations, group activities, and so on.

Diversity includes all the ways that people differ, and it encompasses all the distinctive characteristics that make one individual or group different from another. It is all-inclusive and recognizes everyone and every group as part of the diversity that should be valued. It involves different ideas, perspectives, and values.

Inclusion is authentically bringing traditionally excluded individuals and/or groups into processes, activities, and decision/policy-making in a way that shares power—the answers to questions such as "Have you been invited to the party?" "Were you asked to dance?" "Were accommodations available as needed at the dance?" "Were you included in conversations and idea generation?" and "Was the music you want played considered?" If one is being *included,* the answer is "yes."

We know that to do the critical and impactful work of systems change, we must have an open mind. We must start with a basic understanding of accepting that we do not know all there is to know about any body of work or anyone's lived experiences other than our own in most cases, and more specifically, that we have spent most of our time assimilating cultures to a white*-identified standard of correctness.

Among the questions that public health practitioners should ask include: How do we open ourselves to the work? How do we practice reflective listening that, by its very nature, is deep and personal *and* uncomfortable? Admittedly, listening to others reflect on how our behaviors and our workplaces do not encourage, support, or lead with the intentions of building an equity-based environment—whether intentional or not—is hard work.

Listening for clarity and understanding is a key component in moving toward true systems change. To move toward an unprotected position of vulnerability and to face the truth about ourselves and our roles in our organizations require a willingness to have courageous conversations. To have these conversations means we do not come with our preconceived ideas, agendas, or expectations. Systems are made up of people, and in most leadership positions in our institutions, public health and beyond, those people are white. Even with increased diversity efforts over the past few decades within and across different industries, this has not changed much. In *Diversity, Inc.: The Failed Promise of a Billion Dollar Business*, the author Pamela Newkirk states "the plodding pace of change a half century later makes clear the need to reframe the diversity conversation of recent years from a rosy we-are-the-world ideal to one fired

---

* Morten Group is currently choosing to use "white" as opposed to "White" to describe those who self-identify as such. Those who share this identity do not have a shared experience of being discriminated against because of skin color and, in fact, have historically received benefits based on that skin color. We recognize the many ethnic identities that are currently comprised within this identity (e.g., Irish, Italian, Polish, etc.); however, white supremacy culture has negatively impacted all races and white people particularly through the specific loss of ethnic identity. Race is currently the number one factor, statistically, in how one fares in life, and keeping a small "w" for white and a capitalized "B" for those who identify as Black represents, for us, the opportunity to further name and work to dismantle this systemic power dynamic.

by a mission to combat systemic racial injustice and pervasive delusion about where we stand."[4] Moving past "differences" to the increasingly more transformative work of leading organizations toward a compelling vision of racial justice means addressing the public's health mandate of building healthy communities across the spectrum of oppressive systems experienced by marginalized communities. To address oppression, which occurs when harm is experienced in an unfair, controlling, and abusive manner, it is understood that systems change must go beyond what is performative and superficial for lasting impact.

To move beyond what has been accepted and, in some cases, encouraged for so long requires transformation for system leaders on multiple levels. The diagram in Figure 6.1 indicates the various levels of oppression and how it shows up in our work.

The following is an exercise that practitioners can use to explore the questions that can be elicited from the definitions in Figure 6.1.

> *Explore these questions in small groups to further your understanding of the different levels of oppression. Share some of the highlights of your conversations in a large group setting. Notice any similarities? Any differences? How can you change organizational policies or procedures to create a more equitable workplace culture?*

Individual/interpersonal/internalized: What are some of the attitudes/biases/stereotypes that contribute to the experiences of inequity and oppression in the organization and among those served by the organization? What are some examples of interpersonal interactions that contribute to the experiences of inequity and oppression in the organization and among those served by the organization?

Institutional: How do various institutions (housing, employment, education, media, healthcare, government, religion, family) manifest inequity and contribute to the oppression and inequities experienced by individuals and groups served by the organization?

Cultural: What kinds of images do we see that hold standards of whiteness (e.g., the way that customs, culture, and beliefs operated by those who identify as white are

Individual/Interpersonal/Internalized
✓ Beliefs, attitudes, and actions of individuals that support or perpetuate oppression. It can be deliberate, or the individual may act to perpetuate or support oppression without knowing.

Institutional
✓ The ways in which policies and practices create different outcomes for different groups. The policies may never mention any groups, but their effect is to create advantages for those with privilege and disadvantage for people who have historically been oppressed.

Cultural
✓ Representations, messages, and stories conveying the idea that behaviors and values associated with historically privileged identities are automatically "better" or more "normal" than those associated with historically marginalized identities.

Figure 6.1 Description of levels of oppression.

seen as the standard by which all other groups are compared) as the acceptable and prevailing ideal? How are messages of inadequacy perpetuated by undervaluing cultural practices that may be different than those of the majority population?

ESTABLISHING A READI CULTURE

It is important to note that work to change READI systems is never-ending. We will not arrive at a destination; however, in doing this work, we will have a deeper understanding of what is necessary to be equitable and inclusive, and it is through this practice that we will move toward the desired culture. Practitioners can expect this to take daily practice with incremental change seen along the way; it is important to start this work with that realization as key to its continued success and wins along the way. The following steps help establish an organizational READI culture.

Assume positive intent: To have constructive conversations across differences, embrace a mindset that something good will happen as a result. This requires assuming positive intent from everyone, in that you must consciously choose to believe that people act and speak to the best of their ability and for the benefit of others. By assuming positive intent, we put our own judgments, viewpoints, and biases aside and focus on what the person actually means. This may also mean presuming that others can be responsible for their choices and behaviors and holding them accountable for assuming positive intent from us and others.

Engage in dialogue, not debate: Engaging in a debate (back and forth exchange with contrasting viewpoints) may be counterproductive for promoting inclusion in the workplace. Debates can quickly turn into arguments and result in negative feelings and stalled progress. Instead, dialogue fuels deep understanding and action. Dialogue is open-ended, allowing people to express and learn from one another's experiences, viewpoints, and perspectives. Shared learning is the goal, and it results in deeper connections with people who may be different from us.

Demonstrate cultural humility: To foster inclusion, we must commit to ongoing learning, mitigating bias and inequities; humility; and holding ourselves and others responsible for actions. These are the core elements of cultural humility, defined as a process of self-reflection and discovery in order to build honest and trustworthy relationships,[5] and are critical regardless of one's position of power or dominant/non-dominant group.

Be open, transparent, and willing to admit mistakes: Sharing and deepening understanding of colleagues' experiences at work will help reinforce open and honest communication and cultivate inclusion. Yet, we all can inadvertently make mistakes or say something we regret. We need courage and a personal sense of accountability to admit and learn from mistakes.

Embrace the power of reflective listening: Inclusion requires *really* listening rather than only hearing what someone is saying. In this way, listening requires humility and a willingness to pause and put your own ego, assumptions, and viewpoints aside to reflect on and learn from someone else's experiences. This includes attending to others with empathy by reflecting on what they are experiencing, asking clarifying questions, and gaining a deeper understanding.

Create a trusting, safe, and brave space—where discomfort is okay: Although uncomfortable, engaging in dialogue across and about our differences can accelerate progress—if done correctly. What is deemed safe may look different to an individual with a different cultural background, experiences, and expectations. Sometimes ground rules to "share freely" can mislead individuals to think their viewpoints, opinions, or perspectives will not be challenged. While we all want to feel safe, feeling brave is the way this work gets done. If we are brave, we will be vulnerable, and we will speak up and ask questions in an open and affirming manner that does not derail the conversation at hand.

Commit to having conversations that matter by speaking up to bridge divides: Each of us has a role to play in creating inclusive work environments by (a) starting with an unwavering commitment to having conversations where people can feel valued and respected for their differences, and (b) being willing to speak up as a champion for inclusion in the face of difficult situations or exclusionary behaviors, bias, and discrimination.

By following the previous steps to building an organizational READI culture, public health practitioners can move beyond being bystanders to being upstanders. As far as identities, for most people their inner circle includes people with identities similar to their own. This reflects the ways that our implicit biases are upheld and reinforced. In general, people extend not only greater trust but also greater positive regard, cooperation, and empathy to ingroup members (those who hold shared identities to us) compared with outgroup members.[6] This preference for people like ourselves is largely instinctive and unconscious. Therefore, affinity bias manifests not only as a preference for ingroup members, but it may also require greater trust. In addition to greater trust, greater positive regard, cooperation, and empathy to ingroup members must be offered to outgroup members.

What are the implications of this in the workplace? For example, when a leader assigns responsibility for a high-profile piece of work, to whom do they entrust that responsibility? They will likely offer opportunities to those individuals they trust the most.

Those people, it turns out, are similar to themselves. Because success on high-profile assignments is critical for emerging as a leader, a tendency to favor people like ourselves when assigning stretch assignments leads to self-cloning and promotes homogeneity in leadership. Though not intentional, people who are not like the leader may often get overlooked and left behind. This phenomenon can be especially detrimental in the public health space where many practitioners may work in and serve communities they are not from.

DESCRIBING THE PROCESS AND APPROACH

Morten Group is a multiracial, cross-generational firm that has consciously, intentionally, and thoughtfully built a team of diverse perspectives and experiences; it is important that this READI framework efforts are completed first internally before helping other organizations, which then facilitates systems change specifically embedded within a READI framework.

As discussed earlier in this chapter, organizational change requires commitment and focused intentionality to affect systems change. The need for practical and applied work at a systems level needs strong leadership at multiple levels within and outside of organizations to then impact systems and those served by these systems. Organizations are part of larger systems within public health and abroad, so it is impossible for systems to be transformed without change occurring within organizations for the common good.

Organizational leadership works to support systems change (e.g., moving from a service delivery focus to a focus on policy change, particularly from a diversity, racial equity, and inclusion perspective). Leaders, particularly those in public health, must talk about race and address race equity. To do so is crucial in meeting the mission of their work and serving not just one subset of communities, jurisdictional and otherwise, but all people in an inclusive manner.

An essential element of organizational change is also assessing, in the process of planning, where practitioners fall in terms of our relationships to power in different areas of our work. Often, marginalized communities are negatively impacted by institutions that offer them programs but deprive them of power. The next few pages describe an approach to racial equity work, beginning with facilitating assessments to developing customized training to partnering in the evolution of action planning development.

This approach assists organizations in moving from their current status to the desired state, starting with an assessment of where an organization is/how it is "showing up" to this work, followed by training to make sure all are on the same foundational level. After that, continuing with action planning and deeper training to further address and document an organization's ongoing READI work is key to the overall process.

Assessment

Morten Group employs two major philosophies in conducting assessments and analyzing results in partnership with client partners: a participatory action model for data collection and an asset-based model for data analysis, both of which are used broadly by public health practitioners. "Participatory action" refers to the collection of the data through multifaceted engagement of a variety of stakeholders invested in the assessment process. A participatory action model is vital, as it is the best model through which to understand the opinions and experiences of many different stakeholders at multiple levels.

"Asset-based" refers to a method of analysis emphasizing the strengths and assets of an organization. Instead of working from a standpoint of weaknesses, assets-based analysis operates on the assumption that the opposite of a strength (or asset) is a need, or challenge—defining the path forward not as a series of flaws in opposition to the "right" thing, but rather as the normal issues that arise over the course of an organization's lifetime. These can be reassessed and reimagined for continuous, sustainable growth. This model also works to utilize current strengths to address identified needs, thus presenting a more comprehensive approach to the assessment process overall.

Assessment tools may include the development of qualitative and quantitative tools such as surveys, interviews, and focus groups, as well as review of written documents, including health improvement and strategic plans, annual reports, human resource policies, and so forth. In our assessment process, we recognize four areas that impact organizations: people, programs/projects, places, and policies/procedures. Questions that practitioners can consider in these areas are described in Table 6.1.

TABLE 6.1 The Four Ps for Organizational Change

PEOPLE	PROGRAMS/PROJECTS	PLACES	POLICIES AND PROCEDURES
Are stakeholders engaged at every level (staff, interns, vendors, constituents) to understand experiences and needs? If so, in what ways?	How are each of your programs/projects intentionally addressing inequity?	Are the spaces where your stakeholders work and gather, both physically and virtually, equitable, accessible, and inclusive for all?	Are your policies and procedures intentionally anti-oppressive and equitable?
What are the demographics of stakeholders?	How is cultural responsiveness being approached?	What is the level of accessibility to the following: technology, languages other than English, consideration for neurodiversity, range of motion, and where physical buildings are located, e.g., close to public transportation?	Have you kept a history of how people are being attracted to the organization (staff, interns, partners, volunteers, clients, constituents)?
What is success/satisfaction by identity?	In what ways is resource distribution occurring?		How/where is recruitment taking place (across positions, including staff, interns, board members)?
What is retention and attrition by identity?	Is shared decision-making/community leadership being modeled? If so, in what ways?		Are the job/role requirements and expectations equitable, relevant, and clear?
			How are people developed and supported? How is onboarding accomplished? What ongoing training is provided? Is paid time off equitable? What are the advancement opportunities? Are salaries fair?

Training

Insights, experiences, and recommendations from the assessment are then shared with the organizational leadership in the form of a written report followed by customized training. We emphasize that these trainings are not a "one and done" but a critical step in the organization's racial equity journey to ensure all have been exposed to foundational concepts and definitions. In tandem, this emphasis allows for deep listening of staff, board, and other stakeholders at the organizational level, and then by the nature of this work, impacting the system.

Moving Forward—Action Planning and Monitoring

Figure 6.2 depicts the overall journey described. Among the most critical pieces of continuing the work past the assessment and subsequent initial training is the development of an action plan. This necessary tool provides a guide and a means to monitor progress and manage change. See Table 6.2 for a sample action plan highlighting a specific objective within the plan.

The approach includes advising client partners that the hard work starts after the development of the action plan, as the action plan solidifies and documents what is being done to center change within an organization. As an added resource, the provision of templates to help organizations develop their plans, including defining goals, objectives, and strategies/tasks, as well as helping them answer for themselves the following important questions is key: (a) What are the key areas of focus you are considering for your organizational/departmental plan? (b) What are your concerns about being able to successfully implement your plan? The process of answering these questions in a collaborative manner helps ensure the buy-in of the action plan (once finalized by the governing entity). Ongoing monitoring of the process and a realistic view of progress are essential; in the preceding example, a color-coded system to show levels of progress and completion is used.

Federally Qualified Health Center Vignette

A successful partnership with Erie Family Health Centers (EFHC), a federally qualified health center (FQHC) founded in 1957 as a project of volunteer physicians from

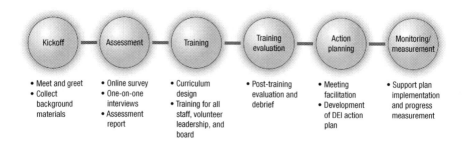

Figure 6.2 Illustration of a racial, equity, access, diversity, and inclusion (READI) journey with client partners.
DEI, diversity, equity, and inclusion.

TABLE 6.2 Sample Action Planning—Objective

Example Goal—Public Health Entity X makes Board of Health, staff, and leadership opportunities accessible to people of color, with a particular focus on accessibility for people of color living in rural areas.

OBJECTIVES	STRATEGIES/TASKS	TIMELINE (WHEN COMPLETED)	LEAD	MEASUREMENT OF SUCCESS	PROGRESS STATUS
PUBLIC HEALTH ENTITY X will create a diverse volunteer pipeline.	1.1: Create culturally appropriate materials and communications for outreach using the input and perspectives of culture bearers	1.1: Q3 202X (to align with next fiscal year cycle)	1.1: Volunteer Manager (VM), Communications and Outreach Manager (COM)	1.1: Culturally appropriate materials, physical and electronic, generated and available to staff and board for outreach	SOME PROGRESS
	1.2: Expand and deepen partnerships with already identified businesses and organizations led or owned by communities of color	1.2: Ongoing	1.2: Regional Philanthropic Officers (RPO), CEO	1.2: Increased presence at gatherings, activities, and events organized by communities of color	SOME PROGRESS
	1.3: Identify, recruit, and retain community members reflective of the regional culture and/or diversity within each public health jurisdiction, region, etc.	1.3: Ongoing	1.3: VM, RPOs	1.3: Potentially four to six individuals per state identified reflecting a broad coverage of public health jurisdiction, region, etc.	COMPLETED

Northwestern Memorial and Erie Neighborhood House is a current example of a public health system entity that is successfully navigating its way in this work. As a client partner, Morten Group has assisted them with a bold endeavor to center diversity, equity, and inclusion within and across all 11 of its community-based health center sites. Morten Group initially partnered with EFHC in 2019 to perform an assessment, develop and facilitate trainings to its then 650+ staff, and subsequently facilitate the development of an internal diversity, equity, and inclusion (DEI) committee. Since then, the ongoing partnership has resulted in the establishment of a diversity, equity, and inclusion plan as well as ongoing additional capacity-building efforts. EFHC is setting an example that can be modeled and customized by other FQHCs and similar healthcare settings. As he was envisioning the ongoing actualization of the health center's work and the ways success can be measured, Lee Francis, MD, MPH, president, and CEO, said, "I will consider the work a success if the language of diversity, equity, and inclusion, if the practices of diversity, equity, and inclusion, and if the understanding of diversity, equity, and inclusion all become part of Erie Family Health Centers' culture, not just for the short term, but for the long term."[7]

As EFHC builds upon 3 years of accomplishments through the partnership —for example, pronoun practice in medical records, DEI committee successes, an onboarding process that includes the health center's commitment and expectations for the values and principles—READI efforts are embraced as the health center's journey continues.

FINAL THOUGHTS

As evidenced in The Equity Center's report "Awake to Woke to Work,"[8] as well as the examples discussed, the road to equity is long and complicated. True systems change requires systems leadership that has a bold vision and an interest in transparency, communication, and collaboration. For this bold vision to be centered, along with the necessary ongoing steps to the systems changes discussed in this chapter, it can take several years with incremental change seen along the way. Even after this period, the work continues. It is never-ending. Specifically in public health, the unlearning and dismantling of inequitable practices, disruption of the status quo, and critical analysis of the root causes of health and social inequities require a systems approach to ensure that this work moves forward. The social determinants of health have never been more relevant, as indicated by the recent statement from the American Medical Association that cites racism as a public health threat.

Understanding that health inequities will continue to heighten and deepen the disparities experienced by historically marginalized communities is a critical first step in this much-needed systems change. As public health practitioners continue to further understand and address health inequities and the role racism has played, it is important that they anticipate barriers that can hinder this work.

Lessons Learned and Barriers to Avoid

Strategies and techniques for effective systems change and systems leadership were discussed earlier in this chapter. Following are some potential barriers and suggestions for moving the work forward that have been learned over time from working with organizations:

- *Treating the work as linear and finite rather than iterative and ongoing.* This work does not have an endpoint and at the same time, is a marathon and not a sprint. Expect and prepare to go through cycles instead of following a straight line.
- *Failing to prioritize intersectionality or believing that the organization's mission, clients, or wins in some areas make additional/ongoing work unnecessary.* Organizational culture is key and is just as important as the quality of programs and service delivery. All must be a focus of the READI journey.
- *Expecting immediate results.* It takes time for change to occur. Acknowledging that process and embracing the need for change can take years.
- *Expecting marginalized people to do all the work.* There must be buy-in and champions across all levels of an organization, without marginalized people expected to do all the work. Diverse teams must be built and supported to do this work within and across organizations.
- *Failing to demonstrate enthusiasm from the top of the organization.* Leaders' enthusiasm can be contagious throughout an organization. When staff hear and see this enthusiasm, it is important that the words spoken match the actions taken.
- *Failing to integrate this work at every level and department organization-wide.* All parts of the organization must be on the READI journey at the same time for true and lasting change to take place.
- *Treating the work as a peripheral consideration or additional/volunteer work rather than central to an organization's mission and embedded in its culture.* This work cannot be tacked on to staff responsibilities without acknowledgment (and ideally compensation or other benefit) of it being in addition to day-to-day roles and responsibilities. This should not be seen as a side project, but something foundational to the overall success of the organization.

Not addressing any one of these barriers can derail progress on building a READI culture. The key is to always come back to the earlier *openings* of seeing the larger system, building relationships that are reflective and interpersonal, and paying more attention to reactive problem-solving and co-creating the future.

To move forward to address systems leadership with clearly articulated, actionable, and equitable practices and policies requires a steadfast commitment to the journey toward systems change. This journey, whether within the public health system for collective impact or other areas and industries, is one that can yield lasting, impactful positive outcomes for all—leaders, those they lead, the communities served, and the individuals impacted.

CHAPTER SUMMARY

This chapter explored steps in leading organizational change to further racial equity, access, diversity, and inclusion (READI) within an organization while addressing positionality/power/privilege at the organizational level. Organizational change is a process that must be grounded in a READI lens. Our organizations need a simultaneous power shift that includes the dismantling of longstanding organizational practices and policies and the elevation of the voices of those who are most often ignored, undervalued, or silenced. Specific leadership strategies can be applied to support these types of change in our organizations. These strategies align with a public health perspective in that they are grounded in community building and collaboration.

Key Messages

- Organizational leadership is the one capacity that *must* be achieved if there is to be any success in systems change in building equitable organizations. Leading with a commitment to consistent communication and respectful dialogue when differences occur while working toward collaboration and communication is fundamental to lasting systems change.
- Understanding the role of power and privilege in this work and being willing to disrupt processes that do not encourage full inclusion of all team members are critical steps toward building teams and accountablity.
- System leaders work across wildly divergent ideas and opinions and build coalitions toward mutual goals. Organizational leaders must motivate team members and secure buy-in and ownership for there to be significant and visible change.
- Becoming a systems leader in building a READI culture in your organization requires a realization that READI systems change work is never-ending. We will not arrive at an end destination; however, we will have a deeper understanding of what is necessary to be equitable and inclusive, and it is through this practice that we will move toward the desired culture.

Tips

- Lead with a commitment to consistent communication and respectful dialogue when differences occur; committing to this while working toward collaboration and communication is fundamental to equitable and lasting systems change.
- Do the difficult work of understanding the role of power and privilege and be willing to disrupt processes that do not encourage full inclusion of all team members; these are critical steps toward building teams that are creative, effective, and accountable.
- Consider wildly divergent ideas and opinions as you build coalitions toward mutual goals. Organizational leaders must motivate team members and secure buy- in and ownership for there to be significant and visible change.

Supplemental Resources

- Microaggressions Are a Big Deal: How to Talk Them Out and When to Walk Away: www.npr.org/2020/06/08/872371063/microaggressions-are-a-big-deal-how-to-talk-them-out-and-when-to-walk-away
- Implicit Association Test: https://implicit.harvard.edu/implicit/iatdetails.html
- Micro Inequities, Attending to the Seemingly "Small Stuff": www.deltaconceptsinc.com/blog/micro-inequities-attending-to-the-seemingly-small-stuff/

- Confessions of a wealthy immigrant— "Model minority" is a myth: www .vox.com/first-person/2017/5/1/15426166/model-minority-myth-immigration
- Toni Morrison on white supremacy: www.openculture.com/2019/08/toni -morrison-deconstructs-white-supremacy-in-america.html
- Responding to Microaggressions in the Classroom—Taking ACTION: www.facultyfocus.com/articles/effective-classroom-management/ responding-to-microaggressions-in-the-classroom/
- 3 Things to Consider When Choosing Between Calling Someone Out or Calling Them In, by Maisha Z. Johnson: https://everydayfeminism.com/2015/03/ calling-in-and-calling-out/
- Gathering Ground, podcasts by Mary F. Morten:

  - Pamela Newkirk, author of Diversity, Inc: https://podcasts.apple.com/us/ podcast/episode-10-pamela-newkirk/id1478561585?i=1000460178919
  - Morten Group, LLC READI Symposium: https://podcasts.apple.com/us/ podcast/episode-19-readi-symposium/id1478561585?i=1000501143672

- Morten Group original document, "Are You Ready?": www.mortengroup.com/ wp-content/uploads/2018/05/MG_Are-You-Ready-to-Do-RE-Work_3.13.18.pdf

REFERENCES

1. Jordan J. *Passion* and *Directed by Desire. The Collected Poems of June Jordan.* June M. Jordan Literary Estate Trust; 1980. http://www.junejordan.net/poem-for-south-african-women.html
2. AMA Board of Trustees pledges action against racism, policy brutality. American Medical Association website. https://www.ama-assn.org/press-center/ama-statements/ama-board -trustees-pledges-action against-racism-police-brutality. Published June 7, 2020.
3. Scharmer O, Kaeufer, K. *Leading from the Emerging Future.* 1st ed. Berrett-Koehler Publishers; 2013.
4. Newkirk, P. *Diversity, Inc.: The Failed Promise of a Billion-Dollar Business.* 1st ed. Bold Type Books; 2019.
5. Yeager KA, Bauer-Wu S. Cultural humility: Essential foundation for clinical researchers. *Appl Nurs Res.* 2013;26(4):251–256. doi:10.1016/j.apnr.2013.06.008.
6. Hewstone M, Rubin M, Willis H. Intergroup bias. *Annu Rev Psychol.* 2002;53:575–604. doi:10.1146/annurev.psych.53.100901.135109.
7. Morten Group. Morten Group, LLC: A Glimpse Inside [Video]. YouTube. https:// www.youtube.com/watch?v=QDgqGMwlnf8. Published November 15, 2021. Accessed November 15, 2021.
8. *Awake to Woke to Work: Building a Race Equity Culture.* ProInspire; 2018. https:// ncwwi.org/index.php/resourcemenu/resource-library/inclusivity-racial-equity/ advancing-racial-equity/1456-awake-to-woke-to-work-building-a-race-equity-culture/file

7

Team and Cross-Sector Leadership: Developing Teams for Systems Change

Jeannine Herrick, Christina R. Welter,
Patricia Moten Marshall, and Samantha Cinnick

CHAPTER OBJECTIVES

By reading this chapter, the practitioner will be able to:

* Describe a framework for developing high-performing, cross-sectoral teams prepared to address systems challenges.
* Describe the five key actions high-performing teams take to address systems challenges.
* Name practical tools that can be used to facilitate team development and encourage teams to engage in the five key actions.

INTRODUCTION

This chapter provides an overview of how we can create cross-sectoral and interdisciplinary teams for systems change work, including special considerations around team development and actions that high-performing teams can take to address systems challenges.

THE IMPORTANCE OF TEAM LEADERSHIP TO SYSTEMS CHANGE

Systems change challenges stem from multiple root causes that no one person can address and no one solution will fix. Challenges like persistent population health inequities stemming from centuries of racial inequality are also unlikely to be solved with any one toolkit, evidence-based practice, or how-to training. Instead, we need multiple perspectives working together over time with a creative, collaborative approach.

We need to build flexible teams with the capacity to step back and examine the existing systems that perpetuate poor health outcomes and then design and implement strategies to dismantle, adapt, or create new systems.

Systems change efforts often require "spanning boundaries," also known as working with and through individuals and groups different than our own[1] to effect population health goals for communities. This includes working laterally, across our public health organizations with multiple branches and departments with categorical funding, and working across sectors, bringing together practitioners from public health, healthcare, education, social services, criminal justice, economic development, and more. Teams comprising individuals who typically do not work together are necessary to dismantle, adapt, or create new systems that support positive population health goals and likely don't share common history, terminology, or norms for how to approach scopes of work and problem-solving. Teams might even have different values related to the systems change challenge. These factors are both why the collective efforts of systems change are challenging, but also why they can result in positive, transformative results. We must ask ourselves, "How do we create cross-sectoral and interdisciplinary teams that are equipped for systems change work?"

This chapter better prepares public health practitioners to consider how we can create and sustain effective, high-performing teams across sectors and cultivate team cultures that are supportive to systems change efforts. We explore how to develop a team that is prepared to address systems change challenges and the actions those teams take to do so. Each section names tools and tips for implementation.

DEVELOPING A TEAM TO ADDRESS SYSTEMS CHANGE

Systems change work can be turbulent, full of both conflict and creativity. Having healthy, high-functioning teams is vital for individuals to thrive during the systems change journey. In this chapter we reference healthy teams, thriving teams, and effective teams interchangeably. While there is no single definition for any of these terms, in a general sense, here is a brief overview of some of the qualities associated with each, keeping in mind they overlap and are not mutually exclusive. Healthy teams have members who genuinely appreciate the contributions of other members and recognize that they are stronger working together than individually. Members have positive bonds with one another and exhibit equal parts listening, asking curious questions, and willing participation. Effective teams have a common vision and articulated shared goals. Members have defined roles and are skillful at navigating disagreements with one another. Finally, members of a thriving team are open and honest with one another and conditions exist in which everyone feels safe and compelled to bring their full selves. Members are mutually invested in the work, and this commitment is reflected in the quality of work collectively produced.

Many of the same principles that are true for building effective teams in general are true for teams focused on systems change efforts that will benefit population health. All effective teams go through developmental cycles of forming, storming, norming, and performing.[2] Additionally, teams focused on systems change will need to ascend to a fifth stage, known as transforming, and develop a keen awareness of which behaviors land on a spectrum from dysfunction to high performance. For example, teams that lack focus, disparage one another, interrupt or talk over one another, and/or are dominated by one or two individuals have dysfunctional characteristics. On the other hand, teams that look forward to spending time together, have aligned motivations and goals that are clear, have healthy debates, and appreciate each other's differences and styles of working have characteristics that lead to high performance.

The first stage, forming, is when teams first come together and is the "polite stage" when we feel good about joining the team, are on our best behavior, and size everyone up to see who and what level of talent is on the team. Individual members during forming are typically driven by the desire to be accepted by others and avoid conflict or controversy (Exhibit 7.1).

EXHIBIT 7.1 Six Community-Building Conversations—A Tool for New Teams

Peter Block presents Six Community-Building Conversations[3] that can be used or adapted for teams that are coming together for the first time, or as they change over time. The use of this tool shows intention and commitment to hear all perspectives at critical times in team development. As team members, when we can participate in these beginning conversations with both our heads and our hearts in alignment and demonstrate respect and appreciation for different forms of expertise, including lived experience, we are setting our team up for success.

Invitation: To what extent are you here by choice? What would you need to feel fully free to choose to be part of this project/team (or not)?

Possibility: What is possible if you are successful (future state, vision)? What inspires you about these possibilities?

Ownership: How do you intend to make this experience valuable/relevant to you/the team/the project/your setting? What support do you need to make this happen?

Dissent: What doubts or reservations do you have? What judgments/assumptions do you have that no one knows about?

Commitment: What are your team agreements about how you work together? What is your commitment to the team/work?

Gifts: What is the gift/strength you bring to this team that you might not fully acknowledge? What is the best use of your gifts/strengths on this team?

EXHIBIT 7.2 Boundary-Spanning Walk-and-Talk

- What brought you to your profession?
- What do you enjoy most about your work?
- What do you wish you were doing more of?
- How do you like to spend your time when you are not working?

Additionally, boundary-spanning leadership highlights "walk-and-talk," a set of simple questions to connect with others that can help team members build relationships (Exhibit 7.2).[1]

For individual members to bring their full selves to the team, the structure of team time together can make a difference. Block explains that some conversations are more difficult than others and advises to start with less demanding conversations and build toward higher risk ones that require a greater level of trust. A link to an implementation guide can be found in the Supplemental Resources list.

The second stage, storming, is a transition stage where members begin to test boundaries to determine what are the rules of behavior within the team. Individual members during storming are driven by gathering information to figure out several considerations, including stakeholder agendas, team member expectations, politics, and what is needed to succeed. This is the important stage for systems change efforts because it is in the storming stage when different ideas compete for consideration. For those of us who are averse to conflict, it can become contentious and feel unpleasant. Even if we as a team feel that we have left the storming phase, the exchange of different ideas at different periods in our team's development can create a storming effect of sorts.

Norming is the stage where we reach consensus on our role and purpose as a team. Clarity around purpose and possible pathways emerge as we clarify roles, responsibilities, and desired behavior. During norming, we begin to work well together as a cohesive team.

Performing, not to be confused with being performative, is when we are in our sweet spot, where work flows and relationships are strong. We work collaboratively, and the group establishes a unique identity. We become interdependent and individual team members function competently and autonomously.

Teams can reach the transformative stage when the outcome of the interactions among team members becomes exponentially greater than the combination of the individual contributions. For example, a coalition in which individuals report back on a regular basis about their organization's contributions toward a common purpose or mission is not transformative compared to collective work focused on co-creation, building one another's capacity, and sharing resources, all in the spirit of creating an alternative reality, a future state. New or enhanced relationships, key insights, and boundary-spanning efforts often lead to transformational opportunities.

Although these stages may seem distinct and linear, the team development cycle of forming, storming, norming, performing, and transforming should repeat over time, especially during systems change work, which is iterative in nature. Team membership may change and the work itself will likely be in a constant state of continuous improvement as ideas are tested and reflections are incorporated.

Overall, to effect change from a systems level, our teams need to develop strong foundations of healthy interpersonal dynamics that can be created by going through the five phases of team development. Excitement related to the cause often brings immediate support for individual and group commitment. However, it is important to dedicate time to building trust with one another and enhance our abilities to address conflict since we will be confronted with multiple perspectives when discussing root problems and potential solutions. A deeper level of commitment and accountability can be achieved when these foundations are secure.

FIVE KEY ACTIONS OF HIGH-PERFORMING TEAMS FOCUSED ON SYSTEMS CHANGE

As our teams iteratively cycle through the stages of development and we monitor our behaviors to ensure we are operating at a high level, then we become ready to take action to drive systems change. Systems change work requires awareness and intentionality to think differently and help others to dream of new possibilities and lean into innovation, while resisting the urge to apply pragmatism; otherwise, we might move too fast and achieve only transactional rather than transformational results. For example, making improvements so that an existing affordable housing program is more streamlined from an administrative perspective is transactional; however, working across multi-sector advocacy groups to create new legislation to convert unused corporate office space into multi-use facilities including new affordable housing options could be transformational. To encourage this way of thinking, there are five key actions we believe that high-performing teams should take to address systems challenges. These include embracing expansive thinking; creating intentional, flexible structure; building and sustaining trust and credibility; appreciating authentic dialogue; and cultivating a learning culture. In this section, we define each key action and provide an overview of how teams can put this action into practice with different tools.

Action 1: Embrace Expansive Thinking

Systems change work is different from project-based work that is focused on solving technical challenges. Instead, adaptive challenges, such as integrating racial equity strategies into an organization's programs and services, require teams that are comfortable working together in a way that embraces expansive thinking, the idea that there are numerous pathways and selected efforts that will evolve and iterate over time. To embrace expansiveness, practitioners should (a) acknowledge that there is not one clear or correct choice, (b) resist external pressures to choose an exact path,

(c) encourage innovation even if it doesn't go as planned, and (d) recognize and celebrate others' comfort with ambiguity. Two ways to help teams think differently so they can embrace expansive thinking that can lead to transformative results include seeking out and listening to diverse perspectives and facilitating team work in such a way that innovative ideas are not dismissed prematurely.

Listening to Diverse Perspectives

Systems change work requires intentionally gathering information from diverse sources, so it makes sense that the teams focused on systems change work would also reflect this. We need diverse teams that are well positioned to span boundaries to tackle public health system change challenges. Diverse representation includes both diverse demographics (e.g., race, gender, age, education level) and diversity of thought (e.g., individuals who think differently than we do and with whom we initially disagree with their perspective). In addition, teams most often have members with varying levels of positional authority. There is no denying that power differentials play a role in team dynamics. Strategies to address this include asking for group consensus to leave hierarchy at the door as part of developing group norms, using a neutral facilitator for meetings where power differentials are anticipated to come into play, and encourage team members to frame their contributions honestly and with consideration toward how positionality and power play a role in how and what they share. Additionally, to protect confidentiality, we can be creative about how we will gather team input on particularly challenging topics. Finally, providing coaching from a neutral party to team members with positional authority can help them develop the skills to support other team members in sharing freely without fear of consequences.

Teams should continuously ask, "Who else should be part of team efforts?" Teams can be fluid and flexible, allowing for different members to come and go depending on the current area of focus. When looking for new team members, invite people as close to the local level as possible and ask community partners for recommendations or nominations of those with lived experience. For example, in federally qualified health centers, there is a requirement that 51% of the board members must be recipients of the centers' services.

Hold Space for Innovative Idea Exploration

To assist team members in exploring new possibilities and prevent them from prematurely highlighting flaws in ideas, we can turn to Edward de Bono's Six Thinking Hats framework.[4] Each hat represents a different type of thinking style and prompts each team member to transcend their habitual patterns of approaching a problem or opportunity. Skilled facilitators within or outside of the team can help members through generative discussions that for a dedicated period of time focus on one of the following areas before moving on to the next: facts, exploration of positive values and benefits, potential risks, intuitive feelings, and creative new opportunities. When team members get off topic, the facilitator can point to an alternative time when that category of input will be received. This is a positive way to allow space for new ideas to be explored.

Action 2: Create Intentional, Flexible Structure

As numerous pathways emerge, systems change teams must create an intentional, flexible structure to explore and maximize new possibilities. Within this structure, as team members, we can take on different roles as priorities shift and different strengths are needed. Additionally, we can share in providing direction, authority, power, and expertise. Four ways we can create this intentional, flexible structure include (a) committing to a shared leadership model, (b) clarifying what our team will accomplish and how, (c) naming team values, and (d) developing a team agreement.

Consider a Shared Leadership Model

Systems change teams should comprise members from multiple departments and/or sectors, depending on the challenge. Typically, a shared leadership model works best whereby rather than having a singular leader, leadership is shared among members, or even a sub group of members. This is advantageous because it allows for the chance to appreciate things that might otherwise be overlooked. Shared leadership also takes advantage of a greater array of leadership strengths within the team. We can learn from how one team leader generates collective enthusiasm for an idea, or how another team leader uses a technique to encourage healing when trust has been broken.

One way to move toward a shared leadership model is to identify the natural leadership styles represented in your team. Goleman, Boyatzis, and McKee present six distinct leadership styles (Exhibit 7.3).[5]

When we consider that systems change work is change work, it is clear that certain leadership styles will be more helpful at certain stages to guide teamwork. For example, as new ideas are formulated, a visionary leader can garner support from stakeholders. As people struggle with doing things in new ways, affiliative leaders can ease tensions and coaching leaders can provide learning supports. Pacesetting leaders are integral in establishing plans to take change efforts to scale. As unexpected emergencies arise,

---

EXHIBIT 7.3 Six Positive Leadership Styles

- Visionary leaders mobilize people with enthusiasm and clear vision and frame the collective task in terms of a grander vision.
- Coaching leaders develop people for the future and help identify their unique strengths.
- Affiliative leaders create harmony and build emotional bonds.
- Democratic leaders build consensus through participation.
- Pacesetting leaders expect excellence and self-direction and strive for a better and faster way.
- Commanding leaders demand immediate compliance and focus on what went wrong. They create resonance by providing clear directions in emergencies, thereby projecting reassurance.

commanding leaders can help provide clear communications for short periods. Being intentional as a team to think through who should lead and when is a sign of a healthy team culture.

Intentionally matching the right talents, skills, knowledge, and experience to specific situations can be a tremendous asset. At times, there may be a gap, and temporarily bringing in someone with that specific capacity can help the team dynamics flourish and the overall work thrive. Much of systems change work is letting go of existing systems and giving up power dynamics that have served specific individuals and groups for sustained periods of time. Moving away from traditional, hierarchical structures of leadership and embracing shared leadership models is a step toward making opportunities for co-creation possible.

Clarify What the Team Will Accomplish and How

Often, teams will know that they need to change a system in order to effectively address an adaptive challenge. Given that there are multiple ways to even define the challenge, it is important to invest effort at the start, and continuously throughout the collective work, to articulate the role of our team and what we are hoping to accomplish. Crafting an aim statement to help ensure that all members of the team are working toward the same common goal that would best address the systems challenge brought forward is a helpful tool. To maintain an intentional and flexible structure, aim statements are never set in stone and can be revisited as often as helpful (Exhibit 7.4).

In addition to having a clear collective aim, teams thrive when there are continuous opportunities for self-reflection and assessment related to team dynamics and effectiveness. Lastly, building in opportunities to recognize and celebrate wins along the journey is also central to being a high-performing team.[6]

Name Team Values

Systems change work requires flexibility, nimbleness, and adaptability; therefore, it would be advantageous if our systems change teams also valued those same core principles. Naming team values when starting this work can help to create and maintain an intentional, flexible structure that will help teams lean into difficult situations. One way to approach naming team values is to ask team members to silently list and rank their 10 most important values that guide their personal contributions. Then, ask members

---

EXHIBIT 7.4 Template for Creating a Team Aim Statement

Complete the following statements as a team:
1. We aim to _____ because _____ for _____ by _____.
2. We will achieve this by _____.
3. Our goals include _____.

to list and rank what they think the top 10 most important values are for the team to advance systems changes related to their challenge. Have them post their top five, and then group them. Facilitate an engaging discussion exploring their rationale for selected values, how they define the values related to the challenge, and what else might be needed to achieve success. Newly established teams might discuss common values during the forming stage of development, but it is helpful to revisit team core values at different points while moving through the other stages of development and as priorities shift or become clearer. Making time and space for teams to explore individual and collective values that acknowledge team members, lived experiences, power, and positionality in the organization or partnership, and are related to equity and how they might play out within the team dynamics is important.

Two instances where revisiting shared values may be useful include making difficult decisions and making the commitment to dismantle old systems to create new ones. When tough decisions need to be made, having stated and agreed-upon values to reflect on can be helpful. As our team moves forward, intentionally facilitating team meetings and work sessions in ways that center team values will ensure that progress is in alignment with intentions. Also, systems change efforts require the critical analysis of existing complex systems, potential adaptations, and new developments. It requires multiple perspectives to shed light on the complexity itself and the underlining assumptions, power dynamics, and normalized conscious and unconscious behaviors so that systems improvement efforts benefit. Teams with shared values around these topics are supportive to systems change efforts. For example, as more public health institutions are more intentionally and directly working to dismantle racism in systems, teams and their stakeholders are faced with challenging discussions, negotiations, and decisions. Having stated values to reflect on provides the foundation needed to move forward in new ways. If we say equity is a core value, then shifting resources away from historical patterns of distribution and investing in new ones becomes necessary, not optional.

Team Agreements

Effective teams continuously ask, "What will help our team thrive?" Team agreements are created in the forming stage and get refined in the norming stage. As different people join the team and others leave, priorities shift and new opportunities emerge. Revisiting team agreements at these transition points is helpful to keep it updated and relevant.

Team agreements create the conditions for success based on what is possible, what is worrisome, and the gifts/strengths shared among the team. They are generated, in part, from the conversations that have taken place among team members. They articulate behaviors that will create an environment that team members need to learn, grow, and achieve desired outcomes.

Team agreements can inspire team members and guide their participation. They should be broad enough to enable team members to create shared meaning and depth. They are concise and easy to remember or reference (fewer than 10). Most of all, they invite personal commitment and accountability (Exhibit 7.5).

EXHIBIT 7.5 Sample Team Agreement

We will:

- Have fun together
- Speak freely and by choice
- Make sure all voices are valued
- Honor our gifts and be aware of our challenges
- Treat each other with respect
- Acknowledge one's privilege and power
- Directly face challenging issues with an open mind
- Be open and flexible
- Strive for a shared vision that enables everyone to contribute
- Foster each other's development through trust and support

Action 3: Build and Sustain Trust and Credibility

The third action high-performing teams take to address systems change is to build and sustain trust and credibility. Stephen Covey explains that trust is a function of character (integrity, motive, and intent with people) and competence (capabilities, skills, results, and how people remember past actions).[7] When trust is established, team members can be vulnerable with each other and maintain a safe space for individuals to bring their full and uninhibited contributions in order to unearth innovative, relevant solutions. This allows for a willingness to take risks, fail sometimes, and then learn and apply lessons to the next iteration,[8] ultimately helping our teams achieve their intended impacts. Perhaps even more critical is that teams build trust and credibility with internal and external stakeholders and partners. Systems change often involves taking something apart that has been serving a purpose and benefiting certain institutions, groups, or individuals for some time. Systems change efforts can fail unless teams are intentional about building trust and credibility internally and externally. To build trust, we can turn to Covey's four cores of credibility, which include integrity, intent, capabilities, and results, and engage in the 13 behaviors of a high-trust leader,[7] which we have included in the Supplemental Resources section.

Action 4: Appreciate Authentic Dialogue

The fourth action high-performing teams take to address systems change is to appreciate authentic dialogue. Creative Interchange is a process that centers Authentic Interacting and Appreciative Understanding to make sure team members feel safe and encouraged to express their diversity of thought so that their viewpoints will be valued. When we create an environment where Creative Interchange thrives, we can most effectively harness the creative power of the group and achieve extraordinary results. Productive conversations require "both/and" rather than "either/or" thinking and acting. Occasionally Creative Interchange will naturally occur in teams but often teams need a process to avoid ineffective communication habits. The four components of Creative Interchange include Authentic Interacting, Appreciative Understanding, Creative Integrating, and Expanding Capacity. In the following, each is briefly described and an example is given for how to use this in a team context over time and as the team progresses in its work.

In the first stage, Authentic Interacting, team members are encouraged to both share with integrity, so that the whole group benefits from new information, and listen with humility, so that team members can learn from one another. Team members feel safe and encouraged to express their diversity of thought.

1. Arrange seats in a circle without tables, laptops, or notepads. Create a list of open-ended questions intended to generate sharing of different perspectives. Build in opportunities to acknowledge those who are sharing and those who are listening attentively.

In the second stage, Appreciative Understanding, team members are intentional about creating an open climate in which differences can be surfaced and people empathize with others and validate their perspective. Ideally, team members appreciate diversity and understand and value what others understand and value.

2. Arrange team members to work in pairs for a short amount of time and switch to other partners until everyone has spent one-on-one time with each member on the team. Ask pairs to take turns sharing and validating. Those sharing should speak to a question set by the facilitator, for example, "What are you most fearful of as this work progresses?" Those in the validating role should identify positive characteristics about the sharing member's viewpoint and delay any negative judgments. At the end of the exercise, each team member should write down key insights and how they understand what each of their fellow team members understand and value.

In the next phase, Creative Integrating, team members grow in their ability to tolerate ambiguity and become persistent in the struggle to create new possibilities.

3. Individually ask each team member to make two columns on a sheet of paper. On the left side, have team members write down a view, belief, or behavior that they initially came to the team with. On the right column, have them write down how they are currently viewing, believing, or behaving something related to the team's challenge. As a large group, ask for members to share and ask other members to acknowledge and validate the stated changes. Group the themes together to collectively see emerging alternatives. Ask the group to consider these collective themes and discuss the positive potential impacts of addressing these together versus individually.

In the last stage, Expanding Capacity, team members are functioning as a collective effort and are able to transform ideas into action to facilitate systems change progress.

4. Arrange seats in a circle without tables, laptops, or notepads. Ask members to state what they have learned from the other members and how it has shaped collective work. Discuss new mutual capacities as a team.

More about this framework can be found in Chapter 5. In this section, we will discuss how normalizing conflict within and across teams and team decision-making can lead teams to meet this fourth action of appreciating authentic dialogue.

Normalizing Conflict Within and Across Teams

Disagreement, tension, and even conflict are normal when working to address complex social issues. It is critical that systems change teams become skilled at facilitating discussions that promote healthy debate versus avoiding conflict or engaging in behaviors that are destructive. Modeling recognition strategies, such as saying, "I really appreciated how you listened so intently to my new idea," may be helpful to reinforce positive communication norms. Similarly, modeling acknowledgments, such as saying, "I thought you were courageous today when you offered an alternative view" or "I appreciated you making an effort to explain a new concept using relatable terms," promotes positive communication dynamics. Additionally, reminding the team of stated team agreements and values can also curb detrimental dynamics and interactions.

Shifting a team mindset to embrace conflict as normal and healthy helps the team function at a high level involving mastering versus managing or avoiding conflict.[8] As teams commit to continuous learning by building in opportunities for reflection and feedback, we should intentionally ask ourselves to assess to what degree we are actively engaging productive conflict and pushing ourselves to stretch beyond our typical emotional comfort zones.

Team Decision–Making

Teams typically experience difficulties engaging in and appreciating authentic dialogue when facing a decision that may involve risk or serious consequences. Risk aversion, fear of intended and unintended consequences, concerns over optics, and pleasing stakeholders can take priority over what is required to change a system. Try asking questions such as "What is the cost of doing what we know doesn't work well?" or "How is playing it safe serving the common goals?" to facilitate discussions about risk. To prevent authentic dialogue from disappearing as decisions arise, discuss beforehand which processes will be used and who will make the final decision. Documenting the process and demonstrating how different perspectives were sought are key for systems change decisions. Not all team decisions are made on consensus. What is important is having agreement on the process upfront to build credibility and trust.

In addition to balancing risk, teams tackling systems change challenges will have to consider many moving, changing parts during the decision-making process. Encourage a team mindset that embraces planning in a way that is flexible enough to accommodate shifting resources and priorities. Mapping out multiple scenarios is helpful for team members to think through pathway options. Commit to asking questions that encourage Authentic Interacting, such as "How far can we go toward implementation without knowing all the parameters for resources?" Questions like this can help keep the team in a flexible mindset that can embrace uncertainty. Adaptive challenges require learning, so framing decisions as "at this point in time" or "at this phase of the work" allows for flexibility, growth, and evolution.[9] However, be careful when using this tactic—avoiding decisions because it is easier or protective from other potential consequences won't lead to transformational results.

Existing systems are also complex and layered with many established structures, processes, and procedures. It can be daunting to begin the work to disassemble them to make room for something better. Teams may struggle to take ownership of decision-making because it is overwhelming. In these situations, it is helpful to step back and first work on questions such as "How are these structures/processes/procedures serving the common goal?" or "Are these structures really unchangeable?"

All the positive communication strategies outlined earlier and in Chapters 5 and 6 are important to be mindful of when decisions feel high stakes. Facilitation should be designed in such a way that all voices are heard. And remember, in systems change work, if the stakes feel high, it is typically because the work is high impact.

Action 5: Cultivate a Learning Culture

The fifth and final action high-performing teams take to address systems change is to cultivate a learning culture, which is described as meaningfully connecting the team's purpose to value learning. A team that cultivates a learning culture encourages and supports members to try new things that may not always succeed; prioritizes constant, frequent, and intentional reflection; and applies learning in order to adapt and redesign work. When a team does this, the goal is not about accomplishing tasks, but rather maximizing learning opportunities to discover the underlying issues holding systems problems in place. To do this, teams focused on systems change will need individual team members to conduct inner work to adopt a learning mindset. Additionally, teams will need to establish group commitment to learn from others, ultimately becoming a learning organization that can use new knowledge and insights to modify its own behavior to make change.

Learning Mindset

We join collaborative systems change efforts as individuals and as organizations typically with the intention of making change by moving toward action. However, joining systems change efforts for the purpose of learning may be the more impactful intention of collaboration. Adaptive challenges require working collectively in ways that support the exchange of ideas for sustained periods of time. While natural human tendencies often lead teams to quickly shift to brainstorming solutions, systems change work demands that we spend extra effort identifying root causes and drivers in deep, analytical ways. This often feels different than the typical way teams function to solve technical challenges. Focusing on ensuring our teams are asking the right questions is what stimulates a learning mindset.

Mutual Learning and Conversational Capacity

Mutual learning is a way that a learning mindset is applied to our communication and relationships with people in our team. It is a way that people interact with each other by asking questions, viewing differences as an opportunity for learning. Mutual learning also accepts that conflict is natural and healthy and will occur when different people advocate for different solutions that cannot all be accommodated.[10] Another way to improve learning among team members is to build conversational capacity, in which the dialogue is non-defensive, safe, and balanced between both parties. In conversations like this, there are equal parts candor and curiosity.[11] This is where teamwork happens best. If we lose candor, team members can shut down. If we lose curiosity, team members can get emotional or "heat up." To do systems change work, teams must be committed to continuous learning-driven communication to gain insight and creativity from and with their partners to see problems and solutions in new ways.

Learning Organizations

As we commit to learning in our teams, the creation and application of new knowledge can be integrated into the cultures of large organizations. Peter Senge describes learning organizations as groups of people who are willing to stretch their thinking so that they can reach beyond typical limits.[12] Teams that value the learning organization perspective explore possibilities, create and try new ways of contributing, and build in plentiful opportunities to reflect and make improvements. "Failing" is normalized as part of the process, and the goal is focused more on learning than it is on specific outcomes. Overall, members of a learning organization work and support each other in their individual and collective learning journey.

There are many tools and approaches that can be used to promote a team to cultivate a learning culture. One tool, O.R.I.D., has been used in multiple public health settings to facilitate collective work for systems change. O.R.I.D. is a facilitation structure that promotes systems thinking to get better results, often through teams. It helps us dig deep into what we know and how we feel before we jump too fast into selecting potential solutions and then subsequently critiquing possible pathways. The structure helps us slow down before making important decisions (Exhibit 7.6).[13]

EXHIBIT 7.6 The O.R.I.D. Method

O—Objective questions such as, "What do we know about this?" At this stage, the group discusses and documents facts, not feelings or interpretations.

R—Reflective questions such as, "How do we feel about this?" Fears and concerns may surface.

I—Interpretive questions such as, "What does it mean for me/you/the team, and so forth?" Potential impacts are discussed.

D—Decisional questions such as, "What are we going to do?"

CHAPTER SUMMARY

Systems change work is a team sport, requiring multiple perspectives and ideas from a diverse group of people dedicated to learning and transformation. Creating teams that can meet those requirements involves taking the time to develop a high-performing team that can focus on the work required to shift from transactional to transformational change. A team built on a foundation of healthy interpersonal dynamics and that can reinvent itself through the phases of forming, norming, storming, performing, and transforming will be strong yet flexible enough to undertake complex and fast-moving systems change challenges. With those team dynamics in place, teams can focus on the five key actions of systems change critical to advance equity: embrace expansiveness; create intentional, flexible structure; build and sustain trust and credibility; appreciate authentic dialogue; and cultivate a learning culture. Resources and materials for developing systems change teams and performing the five key actions of systems change are included in the Supplemental Resources list at the end of this chapter.

Key Messages

- *Intentionality* is required to create and develop cross-sectoral and interdisciplinary teams that are flexible and equipped to dismantle, adapt, and create new systems that will better address persistent population health challenges.
- The team development cycle is not linear and *should repeat over time* to align with the iterative nature of systems change work.
- Instead of striving for teams to avoid conflict, they should instead *embrace* conflict as normal and healthy as transformative work occurs and team members are stretched beyond their typical emotional comfort zones.

Tips

- Frequently step back and ask reflective questions about where the team is in the team development process and where the collective systems change work is in the planning and implementation process, and critically question if additional perspectives would be beneficial, if new or alternative pathways would be helpful to revisit, or if the work is gradually reverting to solving technical versus adaptive challenges.
- Team members should continuously ask themselves if they are curious enough about other team members' ideas and perspectives.
- Reward each other for demonstrating flexibility to encourage a team mindset that can work effectively when the outcome is unknown and parameters, resources, and drivers are changing.

Supplemental Resources

- Tips for Remote Team Success: www.imd.org/research-knowledge/articles/ Leading-virtual-teams-in-times-of-disruption/
- Six Conversations Guide: http://mncampuscompact.org/wp-content/uploads/ large/sites/30/large/2018/06/SIX-CONVERSATIONS-Handout-Campus -Compact.pdf
- *Strengths Based Leadership* Book: www.amazon.com/Strengths-Based -Leadership-Leaders-People/dp/1595620257/ref=sr_1_5?dchild=1&keywords= clifton+strengths&qid=1610241656&sr=8-5
- Team Agreement Template: https://ctb.ku.edu/en/table-of-contents/leadership/ leadership-ideas/team-building/main
- Thirteen Behaviors of High Trust Leaders: www.unthsc.edu/values/ wp-content/uploads/sites/11/13-Behaviors-of-a-High-Trust-Leader.pdf

REFERENCES

1. Why You Should Collaborate Across Boundaries. Center for Creative Leadership website. https://www.ccl.org/articles/leading-effectively-articles/boundary-spanning-the -leadership-advantage/. Published November 18, 2020. Accessed January 15, 2021.
2. Tuckman BW. Developmental sequence in small groups. *Psychol Bull.* 1965;63(6):384–399. doi:10.1037/h0022100.
3. Block P. *Community: The Structure of Belonging.* Berrett-Koehler; 2008.
4. De Bono E. *Six Thinking Hats.* Little, Brown; 1985.
5. Goleman D, Boyatzis RE, McKee A. *Primal Leadership: Unleashing the Power of Emotional Intelligence.* Harvard Business Press; 2013.
6. Langley GL, Moen R, Nolan KM, Nolan TW, Norman CL, Provost LP. *The Improvement Guide: A Practical Approach to Enhancing Organizational Performance.* 2nd ed. Jossey-Bass Publishers; 2009.
7. Covey SR, Merrill RR. *The Speed of Trust: The One Thing That Changes Everything.* Free Press; 2008.
8. Lencioni PM. *The Five Dysfunctions of a Team: A Leadership Fable.* John Wiley & Sons; 2010.
9. Heifetz G, Linsky M. *The Practice of Adaptive Leadership: Tools and Tactics for Changing Your Organization and the World.* Harvard Business Press; 2009.
10. Schwarz R. *Smart Leaders, Smarter Teams: How You and Your Team Get Unstuck to Get Results.* John Wiley & Sons; 2013.
11. Weber C. *Conversational Capacity: The Secret to Building Successful Teams That Perform When the Pressure Is On.* McGraw Hill Professional; 2013.
12. Senge PM. *The Fifth Discipline: The Art & Practice of the Learning Organization.* Crown; 2010.
13. Stanfield RB, ed. *The Art of Focused Conversations: 100 Ways to Access Group Wisdom in the Workplace.* New Society Publishers; 2000.

III

The Process to Lead Systems Change

8

Leading Change Through Partnership: Community Organizing, Coalition Building, and Engaging Nontraditional Partners

Jonathan Webb

CHAPTER OBJECTIVES

After reading this chapter, the practitioner will be able to:

- Identify the principles that underlie meaningful relationships or partnerships, even in the absence of specific grant opportunities.
- Discuss partnership types.
- Detail frameworks and tools for successfully engaging partners.
- Outline strategies and lessons learned from collaborative efforts.

INTRODUCTION

This is a significant time in our nation's history to discuss change and the way public health professionals can and will lead us through it. The country is grappling with an unprecedented pandemic and is coming to grips with how an ugly history of racism has embedded itself in our systems and structures. It is being further challenged by a polarized political climate, civic unrest, the ramifications of prolonged social distancing, and a struggling economy. As a result, we are faced with defining a new "normal." By no means is this list exhaustive—these challenges have arisen recently and build on the many problems and issues already confronting the country.

The public health community has been catapulted into the spotlight. Our leaders are actively responding to coronavirus disease 2019 (COVID-19), leading the calls for racial equity, and helping constituents navigate the side effects of the current environment, including mental and behavioral health issues, lapsed or diminished services for families of children and youth with special healthcare needs, domestic violence, substance abuse, and more. During challenging times and in their aftermath, we have a unique opportunity to learn and grow.

In environments like these, we look for change. As we evaluate the moment and the challenges that came before, one takeaway is that the problems we face are too large for one individual or one organization alone to address. If we are to bring about change and, more specifically, lead change, it will take a collective effort and thoughtful collaboration. This sounds like a simple task and something that public health professionals believe in and aspire to. Anyone who has tried to move systems and partner in developing and achieving a common vision, however, knows that collaborative efforts are more easily said than done. For this reason, this chapter focuses on skills, strategies, and practical frameworks to help you and your organization lead change through partnerships. Collective work with diverse stakeholders is the essential way to build the momentum to create change in our antiquated systems and structures so that the possibility of achieving whole health is available to all people. These new systems will promote community and population health, racial and social equity, and justice.

KEY PRINCIPLES OF PARTNERSHIP

An African proverb says, "If you want to go fast, go alone. If you want to go far, go together." There is an intrinsic urgency to tackling any of the issues mentioned in the introduction that makes a fast-moving effort seem attractive, but hasty, solo efforts generally lack impact and are hard to sustain. We should move with purpose and not delay, but we must couple urgency with a focus on meaningful, long-term impact. This chapter examines partnership types and addresses the nuances associated with building a team, working within a coalition environment, building strategic partnerships, and engaging communities. To start, there are a few key foundational principles that are important across all partnership types. Authentic, honest, meaningful partnerships that have the learning and growth mindset to undertake systems change require: (1) humility, (2) a grounding in equity, (3) strategy, and (4) mutual benefit for all involved.

1. Humility

When leading change through partnership and coalition building, it is essential to approach the work with humility and an understanding that the whole is greater than the sum of its parts. Change leaders must be willing, in some cases, to lead, and in some cases to follow—even to sit on the sidelines and spectate in instances when they are not the best central player or organization for the job. Checking your ego is a must when collaborating with partners or engaging the community in partnership; an organization or individual should never get in the way of the mission. The problems we face are too large for any one organization to solve—thus the need to engage with others. The correct posture is to recognize that common goals as well as a shared vision and out-comes are the glue that brings everyone together and guides the ultimate destination for the group. This should be the most important consideration and should win every time when matched against organizational ego or partner politics.

Humility is important in working with communities for several reasons:

- There are wisdom and key learnings in the rich culture of every community. Entering a community with an inflated sense of self and a lack of appreciation for the community and its leaders makes it much harder to truly learn, listen, and engage with impacted communities with whom you seek to partner. Even well-meaning public health practitioners with theoretical and academic knowl-edge about how to address a given situation may discount the voice of the com-munity and its lived experiences.
- The lived experiences of community members are assets to all systems-change efforts. They provide context and insight that typically will not be reflected in any data set. Community members understand their challenges best and therefore have keen understanding about solutions to their own problems.

Successful community partnerships are based on trust. Demonstrate trust by lis-tening, by a willingness to challenge what you think you know to view things from a different perspective, and by valuing the experiences of the group with whom you are engaging. Entering a community relationship with a paternalistic "I know best" view of the community and a predetermined solution will hinder the trust-building process. This type of arrogance risks diminishing the value of the community's lived experiences and their contribution to the community's solution. It also will negatively impact proj-ect sustainability and could potentially make a solution less comprehensive. A solution developed unilaterally without an appreciation and incorporation of the community's assets will struggle to exist beyond your involvement—it will not live on its own.

2. Grounding in Equity

Partnerships, whether within organizations or in communities, must be grounded in equity, be willing to explore and address the root causes of inequity, and share power (including decision-making). Partnerships need to examine who is and is not at the table to ensure that all relevant voices and stakeholders are heard and valued. A change leader who works collaboratively is responsible for creating an environment with an equitable power dynamic that allows all people who sit at the table to feel that their input is being considered and is balanced. There should be sufficient diversity of thought and culture to prevent the appearance of tokenism—"the practice of making only a perfunctory or sym-bolic effort to do a particular thing, especially by recruiting a small number of people from underrepresented groups in order to give the appearance of sexual or racial equality."[1]

3. Strategy

Leadership expert Lee Bolman said, "A vision without strategy remains an illusion."[2] Determine a thoughtful strategy for the group and a defined logic for requiring the group to assemble before exploring the possibilities around engaging others in the change effort. Coalition building and partnership engagement require investments of time and resources from all parties—if people see these efforts as valuable, they will be willing to take part. Not all coalitions are equal, however, and before inviting people to connect there should be a well-defined reason, one that values the time and energy of participants and is focused on action and outcome. As a group evolves and other stakeholders join, you may modify your strategy—make sure the team is supportive of the changes. Most important, be clear about why the group is meeting and provide a clear plan for how you will move the work forward.

4. Mutual Benefit

Because partnership requires significant amounts of time and energy from those involved, the benefit of participating cannot be one-sided. Organizational partners usually are forthcoming about placing value on their time and will ensure that the benefit received is in line with their mission and business objectives. These conversations are generally set through initial partner discussions and are formalized through a standard organizational process that results in a memorandum of understanding, contract, or the like. For less formal partnerships, at the very least there needs to be clear expectations regarding roles, responsibilities, and resources. If these processes are not a standard part of an organizational partnership, incorporate them into future efforts.

When working with a community, however, conversations about resources, mutual benefit, and business/mission alignment may be neglected. Organizations from outside may assume that addressing the identified problem sufficiently compensates the community for its participation, and that while outside organizations and entities will be paid for their work, community members who partner with these entities will not. In some cases, community members may be supporting project objectives at the same time they work their regular jobs. An initial conversation with community supporters regarding compensation, expectations, and roles will help define mutual understanding and avoid the appearance of exploitation. True community partnership means sharing power, knowledge, credit, and resources. Further, the focus of every project should be to make certain that as much of project dollars and resources as possible stay within the community and that organizations that receive funding to work with communities are given the latitude to implement the projects they deem necessary for meaningful impact. Often, conveying this flexibility may relax the definition of "evidence-based." Community solutions may not have the resources to undertake the evidence-based rigor our field expects, but their results are undeniable. One way to address the root causes of inequity and underlying issues related to disparate outcomes is to ensure that resources such as job creation and procurement and contracting are invested in communities.

The next section discusses the types of partnership frameworks that support collaborative work. The specific partnerships highlighted feature community organizing with elements of community-based participatory research (CBPR) and coalition building. In the community organizing example, components of CBPR related to sharing power with stakeholders were used, but the focus was not on research in the traditional sense. Partners gathered information and worked alongside the community, but not for the purposes of scientific data collection in its purest form.

PARTNERSHIP FRAMEWORKS

1. Community Organizing

In 2010, as division manager of community health for the City of Evanston's health department, I was tasked with identifying programs to address the city's poor health outcomes related to chronic illnesses such as diabetes and obesity. There was a modest grant opportunity ($5,000) from the state of Illinois for a walking program focused on women that had a reasonably straightforward program design and seemed like a worthwhile low-touch engagement. The city budget was tight, so we knew from the outset that the program had to be mindful of costs and creative in its approach. We set out to offer this program to 50 women, and in the first year served 500. The second year, we intended to enroll 500 women and instead served over 1,000. Women Out Walking (WOW) operated in Evanston for approximately a decade, received national recognition with the Council of Mayors Livable City Award, was offered at no financial cost to the city or program participants, and accomplished more than improved health outcomes. WOW was one of Evanston's most successful public health programs[3]—here is why.

Our approach used two frameworks that were fundamental to the strategy—community organizing and CBPR. In the words of Beckwith and Lopez at the Center for Community Change, community organizing is "the process of building power through involving a constituency in identifying problems they share and the solutions to those problems that they desire; identifying the people and structures that can make those solutions possible; enlisting those targets in the effort through negotiation and using confrontation and pressure when needed; and building an institution that is democratically controlled by that constituency that can develop the capacity to take on further problems and that embodies the will and the power of that constituency."[4] CBPR "supports collaborative interventions that involve scientific researchers and community members to address diseases and conditions disproportionately affecting health disparity populations."[5] This research recognizes the strength of each partner and community members and supports collaboration in all aspects of the project, from needs assessment to community-level interventions and even evaluation. "The community is involved in the CBPR program as an equal partner . . . and helps ensure that interventions created are responsive to the community's needs." One of the goals of CBPR is to "establish sustainable programs that improve health behaviors and health outcomes in health disparity populations."[5]

These frameworks were especially important in building the WOW program because if this work was to be for the community, it had to be built with community input. "Community," for purposes of this project, was Evanston women ages 30 to 55. We began by engaging a subset of women from the community to provide insight, make decisions, and assume a leadership role in building WOW. They evolved into a planning committee of approximately 30 diverse stakeholders selected for their connections to the community, the populations they represented, and their roles as gatekeepers, trusted community resources, and influencers within their spaces. Through a series of conversations, the committee set expectations for commitment of their time, for the program and for decision-making. This was their effort—the health department was merely a conduit through which to leverage municipal support.

Beyond respectfully engaging this group as partners, the department's most important actions were listening and learning. Through our discussions, we learned that although the city viewed this as a program for improving health, the planning committee envisioned this as an unprecedented movement to engage, connect, and empower women in the community. Building this shared vision deepened the women's sense of community. Engagement in the process was priority number one, and the programmatic benefits, although vital, were secondary; we viewed WOW through the lens of engagement and connection.

The planning committee helped consider how to recruit participants, build teams, select communication tools, and so on—the women were involved in every aspect of program design. We engaged Evanston's business community to underwrite additional items the committee identified, and businesses were motivated to support this effort and receive exposure among this group. We added elements to the program, including regular sessions on financial literacy and healthy cooking that the committee identified as important components of building community and advancing toward true health. Committee members recruited participants, assisted with program logistics, and led programmatic areas. As owners of the program, they contributed to its initial success and were responsible for its longevity.

WOW provided the opportunity for women in the community to launch and promote business services among themselves and created a long-term relationship between WOW participants and the health department. For years after the program launched, WOW women engaged in health department efforts unrelated to WOW, served on committees, and attended city council meetings to advocate for services and their community.

Benefits of this community-organizing approach include:

- Trust and a strong relationship built with the community that began with WOW and extended into other city operations.
- Insight gained from the community's involvement that directly contributed to the success of the program, including information on how best to meet community needs and how to creatively implement program offerings.
- Enhanced outcomes from co-creating with community partners.
- Community buy-in; members of the planning committee were trusted community ambassadors for the program and owned its success.

Key Considerations in Getting Started

1. Spend time with the community before engaging in a project. Focus on building relationships, understanding community needs and community history, and identifying the trusted community gatekeepers.

2. Develop an initial vision and strategic plan for the program and the partnership.
3. Articulate a clear reason for community outreach.
4. Be thoughtful and clear about demonstrating that you value the time of community members with whom you work.
5. Consider which actions can lead to community benefit and improved outcomes by partnering in the work. What is the added value of this work?
6. Think about the extent to which the perceived benefits and improved outcomes are already being achieved by another effort or initiative. If others are doing similar work, how might your work complement what already exists?
7. Engage partners in developing a shared vision and strategic plan. Be willing to adapt the vision and plan as needed. Reflect on how your organization will signal willingness to change direction based on community insight.
8. Acknowledge that the community is an asset and find ways to highlight and leverage the natural strengths and talents that exist within the community.
9. Show humility in your work with the community.
10. Determine how to share power with your partners, elicit their input, and co-create with them.

2. Coalition Building

Coalition building, or collaborating with multiple entities to lead systems change, is an exciting and worthwhile endeavor filled with possibilities. Groups are generally self-energized and want to leverage their collective power for the good of the shared mission. Without appropriate planning, groundwork, and framework, however, it can be challenging to achieve action and get a group moving in an agreed-upon direction.

Here are some essential steps to help ensure that you set the stage for building a successful coalition:

- At the start, spend time with the group to outline a vision and mission statement, something that defines the group's purpose.
- Through skilled facilitation, identify specific goals for the coalition—what you expect to accomplish. The Agile facilitation approach[6] walks participants through a discussion on current and future states (where things are now and where the group would like them to be), which helps the coalition build actionable goals to connect the dots to impact. Although Agile is a preferred method, use any facilitation method (e.g., Technology of Participation[7]) that helps identify actionable goals. Skilled facilitation will create space for a generative process that engages everyone in developing goals. Carefully design meetings to prevent vocal coalition members from exerting more influence than quieter members who contribute less to the conversation.
- Identify and understand what resources and efforts exist within the coalition to advance your goal. The focus should be on expanding or scaling up efforts that are succeeding, not on duplicating existing work, which is a waste of time, energy, and resources.
- Establish short-, medium-, and long-term milestones so that you can chart a course to success and celebrate short-term wins. Recognizing small victories is an

important way to build and maintain momentum when tackling long-term problems. These celebrations help to motivate and keep members engaged.

- Ensure that coalition members know their individual and organizational responsibilities. All participants should understand what value they bring to the table and what portion of the goal they should address.
- Communicate using a variety of modalities (e.g., texting, Zoom meetings). Face-to-face communication is always best for relationship building but is not always possible. Establish regular times for meetings and other communications; meetings should include check-ins as well as updates. Respect coalition members' time and other commitments by being mindful of how much you communicate and how often you convene. The coalition should determine preferences for communication type and frequency.

March of Dimes—A Case Study

As CEO of the Association of Maternal and Child Health Programs, I was privileged to participate in and, in some cases, lead collaborative efforts with organizational and community partners. More recently, I served as co-chair for the March of Dimes Mom and Baby Action Network's Dismantle Racism and End Unequal Treatment Work Group, a coalition. This was a new cross-sectoral partnership focused on identifying structural and institutional policies that produce inequitable outcomes and on implementing change efforts that positively impact birthing people and their infants.[8] The success of these efforts has yet to be determined, but the coalition is carefully laying the foundation to foster meaningful change.

The work group comprises 30 to 40 national and local organizations that are committed to this work. They include traditional partners—such as national nonprofit public health organizations, community-based organizations, and relevant governmental agencies—and nontraditional partners—such as provider groups or organizations that represent provider groups and funders. We anticipate expanding to include corporations, payers, and other organizations or governmental agencies that work directly with key elements of the social determinants of health, such as housing, criminal justice, and education. In the current social climate, racism and unequal treatment are very visible topic areas—many coalitions, work groups, and partnerships are being formed to address these problems. This is a positive thing, given the long struggle to confront the country's history of racism, segregation, and discrimination. The challenge is to distinguish the work group from other coalitions, to demonstrate value, to respect the group's time and commitment by being action- and results-oriented, and to not duplicate efforts.

At the outset, we spoke with participants about aligning to a coalition strategy and shared goal. We also determined how to measure attainment of the goal, so that as we evaluate the potential benefit of a particular activity we do so against the backdrop of how the task gets us closer to achieving that goal. There are many worthwhile efforts to engage in, and we want to be certain the ones we select not only have impact but also leverage the coalition's abilities and benefit from the attention of these valuable organizations. We are beginning to talk about current state versus future state (see the earlier Coalition Building section) to help us align to the areas the coalition should focus on.

We used the Results Based Accountability (RBA) approach because of its action-oriented design and focus on starting with the end in mind and working backward. The method is data driven and allows for transparent decision-making; it also helped us determine which partners, given their expertise, would take ownership of various aspects of the solution.[9]

The racism and unequal treatment work group is in its infancy, but we are energized about the process we are embarking on and look forward to providing updates on the outcomes of this worthwhile activity. The excitement about our potential is due in large part to how we are approaching this work. Group convenings focus on more than topic discussions; we also discuss actions to turn the curve and improve the lives of and positively impact those we serve and represent.

Frameworks Summary

Having a strategy and approach to collaborating that includes meaningful and thoughtful engagement are essential whether you are building a coalition or organizing in the community. Engagement of any entity should value their contribution, welcome their input, and provide them with a clear expectation of everyone's role in executing an agreed-upon plan. Coalition-building may include impacted community members but typically incorporates organizations that work on a given issue or organizations that represent the community. Community organizing is somewhat more involved and takes more effort to engage individuals, understand historical context, build trust, and mobilize those who have been marginalized. Whether you are engaging in community organizing or working through a coalition, the hard work of collaborating with your partners is required. The approaches outlined earlier will ensure at a minimum that partners are aligned on what they are addressing and why and working together toward a goal.

As you think about who to engage with, it will be worth engaging partners that have a direct impact or influence on the issue at hand, but have typically not been engaged in solution development: the nontraditional partners.

NONTRADITIONAL PARTNERS

The social determinants of health are the conditions in the places where people live, learn, work, and play that affect a wide range of health and quality-of-life risks and outcomes. They have been the focus of public health policy, advocacy, and programming efforts for decades.[10] Health influencers in areas/sectors/industries that we would not typically identify as part of the "public health family" are nontraditional partners and are critical for achieving impact on these social determinants of health. For instance, when thinking about public health, we might call to mind health departments or community organizations doing community education, or in some cases, clinical providers.

We do not typically think about how a partnership with an education, housing, or criminal justice entities (all of which play major roles in the social determinants) might impact the public's health. To lead systems change, we must be intentional about engaging nontraditional partners.

Corporate entities, for example, employ our constituents and are considered nontraditional partners, but because they determine internal health benefits, can offer a livable wage, and can impact the environment around them, they are important partners in improving public health. Other nontraditional partners have the potential to impact housing conditions, education, and so on. Our collaborative work should expand to include these nontraditional partners to ensure comprehensive and sustainable systems solutions to achieving optimal health outcomes.

We should work with these partners in the same ways we work with our traditional partners, although nontraditional entities may require additional effort to attain their buy-in. This is known as "identifying the value proposition" for a specific collaborator. Remember that these nontraditional partners generally have different metrics of success or decision-making priorities than in public health. Well-meaning corporate entities need to consider their bottom line, board of directors, or shareholders as factors in deciding whether to partner. The good news is that many nontraditional partners already think of themselves as stakeholders in public health, and this social consciousness is motivating them to discern how best to support the health of their employees and communities. They also may be able to serve as financial resources and therefore partners in innovation.

To identify potential nontraditional partners, take a creative look at the challenge before you. Examine its root cause as well as other contributing factors. Determine who is impacted by the issue or has a role in contributing to its solution. Consider all stakeholders and players in the system that can effect change, and then determine who you have not meaningfully engaged. That may be your nontraditional partner.

The American Diabetes Association—An Example of Nontraditional Partners

While at the American Diabetes Association (ADA), I led its national efforts around strategic partnerships. In 2016, the ADA wanted to create awareness of diabetes and people's potential risk. Approximately 88 million Americans live with prediabetes and more than 84% of them are unaware they have it.[11] One of the products the ADA uses to help bend the curve of those living with prediabetes—to prevent prediabetes from becoming diabetes—is the diabetes risk test. The risk test is a 97% predictor of diabetes risk. It is not a diagnostic tool but rather a potential flag to encourage test takers to follow up with a physician. The risk test was promoted through the ADA website, social media, and at health fairs. At best, several hundred thousand people took the test each year—a good number, but hardly representative of the 88 million Americans living with the disease.

Through several months of relationship building with an electronics company (meeting to understand shared values and priorities, making connections with leaders within business units, brainstorming solutions, meeting executive leadership, and so on) and several years of relationship building with a well-known retailer, we determined that these two organizations had the potential to amplify the reach of our risk test into virtual and local communities. Although they were motivated by the ability to improve the health of their customers, both companies were launching new corporate health initiatives, and an association with the ADA provided them with credibility and could impact their bottom lines and market shares. We looked creatively at these potential relationships and identified ways to support each other's goals.

Our creativity was rewarded. Our corporate partners earned credibility, the ADA embedded its risk test into the digital platform of one partner, and the other partner allowed us to distribute our information in all their stores four Saturdays a year and to include the test on their digital customer sites. Our first partner's digital platform yielded 550,000 risk tests in 5 weeks. Our second partner, the retail company, gave us store exposure to nearly 100 million customers, of whom one million took the test.

We spent significant time cultivating relationships with these nontraditional partners and understanding the mutual benefit this relationship could provide. We needed to maintain the integrity of our brand and the science, so we scrutinized our partners' reputations and the way we administered the program. Ultimately, these relationships vastly increased our reach, allowing us to engage more people and alert them to their potential diabetes risk.

To support nontraditional partnerships, some funding mechanisms extend beyond traditional governmental and foundation sources and encourage creative public/private partnerships. Social impact bonds, "Pay for Success" models, and social venture capitalists, for example, incentivize new types of partner relationships and help accelerate public–private partnerships through "contracts among a public-sector body (such as a government agency), a private financing intermediary (sometimes known as a social impact bond issuing organization) and private investors, in which the public-sector body agrees to pay for improved social outcomes. These improved social outcomes are to be achieved using funds provided by the private investors."[12] These models have been applied with some success, including in the Massachusetts Juvenile Justice Pay for Success Initiative (PFS).

The Massachusetts Juvenile Justice PFS "is a $28 million partnership between Roca [a Massachusetts-based nonprofit working with urban young adults], the Commonwealth of Massachusetts, the intermediary Third Sector Capital Partners and a host of private investors. Through the project, Massachusetts criminal justice agencies refer high-risk young men to Roca on a monthly basis, and Roca's success in reducing incarceration and increasing employment with these young men is measured by an external evaluator. The private funders cover 85% of Roca's costs and assume most of the financial risk upfront, and they would be repaid by the Commonwealth only if the projected incarceration reduction outcomes are met. Given the high cost of incarceration ($55,000/year per person) and Roca's demonstrated success in reducing re-offending, the project's financial benefits for Massachusetts residents are expected to be substantial. At the project's target impact of reducing incarceration by 40% the project would generate $21.8 million in budgetary savings, and at a 65% reduction the project would generate $41.5 million in gross budgetary savings."[13]

Here are some tips for building relationships with nontraditional partners, key questions to consider, and funding strategies to explore.

Tips for Building Relationships With Nontraditional Partners

- Research the companies/potential partners in your area to generate a list of prospects (and the point of contact) you would like to engage.
- Host meetings or events to meet them; share your priorities and learn theirs. This can be a large event, such as a summit on a specific topic area, or it can be a meeting with one company or a small group of companies.
- Network. Attend gatherings that prospective partners host or attend, such as chamber of commerce meetings.
- Once connected, schedule time to discuss shared goals. Take the opportunity to brainstorm. Allow partners to build with you and get excited about the possibilities of working together.
- Find opportunities to connect with each other by including partners in your events or attending theirs. Relationships take time.

Key Considerations for Working With Nontraditional Partners

When considering whether or not to work with nontraditional partners, consider the below questions for each potential partnership.

- Why are you interested in working with this nontraditional partner?
- What value proposition do you offer? What is theirs? Is this relationship mutually beneficial?
- Is there reputational risk with this association? What guardrails, protections, or firewalls will mitigate this risk?

Funding Nontraditional Partnerships

When working with nontraditional partners, consider the below strategies to assist in identifying funding for these efforts.

- Enroll in educational opportunities to learn to identify and secure funding. Organizations like Foundation Center and Chronicle of Philanthropy offer good resources.
- Consider purchasing access to grant prospecting services such as Foundation Director and Foundation Center. Or employ a professional fundraiser or consultant.
- Produce a business/project plan that clearly details your budgetary needs, priorities, and opportunities for partnership. Clarifying these priorities and opportunities will help you identify prospective partners. If you want to engage people where they are with local programming, look for an established vehicle or

partner already working with your desired population with which you can work to ensure success.

- Spend time with nontraditional partners to identify innovative and unique solutions to challenges. Create an environment where these types of new solutions can be appropriately explored and not dismissed because they may seem to be too radical or less likely to be funded through typical means.

CHAPTER SUMMARY

Our nation is struggling with two pandemics: COVID-19 and structural racism. The public health workforce is being challenged to provide leadership in ways that may be novel for some practitioners, and the issues they face and the outcomes they desire are beyond the scope of one organization, agency, or municipality. To bring about desired change and achieve the shared goal of sustained and equitable health, meaningful and strategic partnership is paramount. This chapter explored strategies and case studies pertinent to coalition-building, community organizing, and community partnership. The approaches are models of how to lead collaborative efforts with humility, respect, and purpose. They emphasize the importance of valuing community insight and community assets in achieving the most comprehensive and sustainable outcomes possible.

Leading change through partnership is not easy, but if done with care it can yield great benefits. Those who are most successful will be bold, creative, innovative, and resilient. Engaging with others to achieve a common goal can be simultaneously exciting and frustrating, and it is important to focus on the impact the partnership can have and to remember that partnering entities are equally focused on positively impacting their constituents. It may not be easy work, but it is worthwhile. Good luck!

Key Messages

- Partnership must be genuine and move at the speed of trust.
- Partnership should be thoughtful and intentional.
- Planning is your friend and good facilitation will help to move things along.
- Value each group's contribution and acknowledge everyone's contribution.

Tips

- Remember that partnering with trust will require patience, a willingness to have the project follow a potentially different path to get to the desired outcome. Be willing to learn about others' experiences even if these experiences challenge what you think you know about the group you are serving. Value the lived experiences of your partners.
- Take time to map out a proposed strategy but be willing to have it change as your group becomes more engaged. Think through who needs to be involved and

why. Think about what value each group brings to the conversation. Set realistic expectations. Value the group's time by planning meaningful meetings with agendas and committing to action items that show progress.

- Invest time in setting the group up for success. Spend time building your facilitation skills or bring in a trained facilitator to ensure everyone is appropriately engaged and contributing to the discussion.
- Look for ways to have everyone's contribution valued and recognized. Share leadership, share recognition, and share power.

Supplemental Resources

Community Organizing

- Community-Based Participatory Research
  - www.ncbi.nlm.nih.gov/pmc/articles/PMC2774214/
  - https://bmcpublichealth.biomedcentral.com/articles/10.1186/s12889-018-5412-y
  - www.advarra.com
  - www.nimhd.nih.gov/programs/extramural/community-based-participatory.html

Coalition Building

- Results-Based Accountability
  - http://raguide.org/2-1-what-are-the-basic-ideas-of-results-based-decision-making-and-budgeting
- Agile Facilitation
  - https://agilebacon.com/twelve-awesome-interactive-facilitation-techniques-for-agile-teams

REFERENCES

1. Hahn H, Felzien L, Xu F. Tokenism in patient engagement. *Fam Pract.* 2017;34(3):290–295. doi:10.1093/fampra/cmw097.
2. Bolman LG, Deal TE. *Reframing Organizations: Artistry, Choice and Leadership.* 6th ed. Jossey-Bass; 2017:205.
3. Evanston CO. 'WOW'—Women Out Walking. *Evanston Now.* https://evanstonnow.com/wow-women-out-walking/. Published March 13, 2010. Accessed February 20, 2021.
4. Beckwith D, Lopez C. *Community Organizing: People Power From the Grassroots.* Introduction to Organizing – Center for Community Change. https://comm-org.wisc.edu/papers97/beckwith.htm. Accessed February 15, 2021.
5. Community-Based Participatory Research Program (CBPR). National Institutes of Health: National Institute on Minority Health and Health Disparities website. https://www.nimhd

.nih.gov/programs/extramural/community-based-participatory.html. Updated October 2, 2018. Accessed February 20, 2021.

6. Badgley M. Twelve Awesome Interactive Facilitation Techniques for Agile Teams. Agile website. https://agilebacon.com/twelve-awesome-interactive-facilitation-techniques-for -agile-teams. 2021. Accessed February 20, 2021.

7. About the Technology of Participation (ToP). Institute of Cultural Affairs website. https://www.top-training.net/w/privateevent/. Accessed February 20, 2021.

8. Mom and Baby Action Network. March of Dimes Foundation website. https://www .marchofdimes.org/professionals/mom-and-baby-action-network.aspx. Published 2021. Accessed February 15, 2021.

9. What are the basic ideas of results-based decision making and budgeting? RBA Implementation Guide website. http://raguide.org/2-1-what-are-the-basic-ideas-of-results -based-decision-making-and-budgeting. Published 2014. Accessed February 15, 2021.

10. NCHHSTP Social Determinants of Health: *Know What Affects Health*. Centers for Disease Control and Prevention website. https://www.cdc.gov/socialdeterminants/index.html. Reviewed December 19, 2019. Accessed February 15, 2021.

11. Prediabetes—Your Chance to Prevent Type 2 Diabetes. Centers for Disease Control and Prevention website. https://www.cdc.gov/diabetes/basics/prediabetes.html. Reviewed June 11, 2020. Accessed February 20, 2021.

12. Lane MJ. *Social Enterprise: Empowering Mission-Driven Entrepreneurs*. American Bar Association; 2012.

13. Outcomes Based Funding. Roca website. https://rocainc.org/work/pay-for-success. Published 2021. Accessed February 20, 2021.

9

Articulate the Root Challenge: Using Systems Thinking to Understand the Problem Before Defining Solutions

Christina R. Welter, Eve C. Pinsker, and Kristen Hassmiller Lich

CHAPTER OBJECTIVES

By the end of this chapter, the practitioner will be able to:

- Distinguish between a technical challenge and a complex, systems challenge.
- Explain why it is important to develop a collective understanding of complex challenges and use this as a foundation for deciding how to address inequity and create more enduring change.
- Define systems leadership and systems thinking and their role and importance in addressing today's challenges.
- Define systems science and its various approaches.
- Articulate how to unpack complex challenges using tools that facilitate this process.

INTRODUCTION

Public health too often focuses on technical problems and not the root causes of persistent unjust and unequal population health outcomes. In addition, as we rush to solve problems, public health practitioners sometimes propose solutions before there is clarity, creating less effective response systems. This chapter describes processes and tools that help to identify and unpack complex issues to obtain shared agreement on the root of a problem and develop a more resilient vision for the future.

THE IMPORTANCE OF PROBLEM DEFINITION TO SYSTEMS CHANGE

Systems leadership is needed now more than ever. Coronavirus disease 2019 (COVID-19) has exacerbated health inequities stemming from longstanding structural and systemic racism. Latinx, Black, and Native American populations have greater COVID-19-related hospitalizations and fatalities compared to their White counterparts.[1] Public health agencies and their partners have had an opportunity to treat COVID-19 as a systems challenge, but response has depended on how key stakeholders defined COVID-19. Considering COVID-19, a variety of questions have been asked that shape action. How you define questions shapes outcomes. Consider two options, both focused on contact tracing: (a) What is the best way to use contact tracing resources to reduce COVID infections? (b) Recognizing that disparate outcomes in COVID-19 are due to historical racism and structural inequity, how can we use contact tracing resources to build capacity in the community to reduce disparate outcomes?

The discipline of public health is challenged with both new and ongoing complex, adaptive problems such as COVID-19 and health inequities. Addressing complex challenges requires systems thinking to consider context, gather diverse perspectives, and explore the multiple interacting root causes operating in an unstable environment. A front-end understanding of the challenge can open the problem definition and uncover what needs to be questioned and investigated rather than letting a pre-emptively defined decision about the problem drive the intervention. The result can lead to an even more generative and positive vision of the future and to fundamental systems change.

Problem definition is a vital early step to undertaking systems change. This chapter discusses why complex problems are so challenging and why public health practitioners need to lead a process to define and explore—versus decide and solve—these issues. To understand these systems issues, we share a process using systems thinking tools that can help us embrace inquiry and diversity, create a shared definition of the challenge, and begin to co-create a more innovative vision for the future and strategies to achieve it.

COMPLEX PROBLEMS AND WHY PROBLEM DEFINITION MATTERS IN SYSTEMS CHANGE

To undertake systems change, we need to consider why complex problems are so challenging. At the core, complex problems show incongruences or gaps between alternative visions of what is happening and/or what is intended to happen. This incongruence is often based on different perspectives and values about what the problem actually is and what is causing it, with the predominate definition often weighted toward those individuals or groups with power and resources. For example, throughout COVID-19, resources are often directed toward "accessible" testing and vaccination, with wide variation in actual "accessibility" across individuals. In addition, we often assume we all have the same definition of what "the system" is and how it operates. Understanding these perspectives and power disparities, and gathering multiple diverse perspectives (rather than jumping to conclusions and solutions that most easily come to mind) can help us explore novel and long-term effective approaches and even redefine "the system" itself, rather than stop at interim, short-term fixes.

Complex problems are challenging for at least three reasons. First, one of the hallmarks of complex problems is we often have different perspectives and worldviews about our shared environment. These worldviews shape and define our perception of the problem and why the problem exists. Our values, lived experiences, and expertise (e.g., disciplinary training, what we have seen/worked on) drive our thinking and determination that our views are correct. We then tend to rush to consensus before embracing diversity and what would be a novel path forward, and we do not ask what the problem is or how it is defined. We make assumptions and generate solutions that allow the problem to persist because they are misaligned with system structure or fail to address root causes. The implications of not questioning our initial assumptions are severe. By focusing on only surface-level challenges, our impact remains limited, whereas addressing root causes may address the structural and social determinants of health that result in persistent sub-optimal outcomes and inequity.

The second reason complex problems are challenging is how we define "the system" itself. For example, how do we define our public health system? Does it include only governmental agencies? Healthcare, health-oriented, or social service agencies? Who is not included and why? The definition of a system is something we as humans construct, and we need to broaden how we think about "the system" producing outcomes we want to change. It includes

- its elements, that is, all the parts that make up the whole;
- the links between the parts, that is, the processes and interrelationships that hold the parts together in view of the whole; and
- its boundary, that is, the limit that determines what is inside and outside a system.[2]

Different people have different perceptions of how a system is defined. What and who are in the system? What are its boundaries? Who is included and who is not? Is the problem hyperlocal, regional, national, or international, or is it all of these? Who gets to decide and how? Is the focus on action or definition? And what matters most? For example, we often focus on what systems do or should do instead of what they contain or how their structure produces outcomes we want to change. How we define the system itself matters, since it determines what is relevant to an inquiry and what is not and shapes what is possible and what is not to address it.

Finally, and probably most importantly, we need to acknowledge and question *who* makes decisions about what is "inside" and what is "outside" of the system. That is, who has influence, resources, and power in defining and choosing pathways to address complex challenges. Whose voices are loudest? Who is heard and seemingly valued the most? Which voices are most likely to influence the decisions and why? How can we build the kind of power that successfully challenges existing influence and authority? Addressing health equity, for example, requires that we deeply examine who is making decisions and for whose economic advantage (and acknowledging the connections between who benefits and how these decisions are made). Until recently in public health, these decisions have rarely included or valued people with lived experience of health disparities.

THE ROLE OF LEADERSHIP IN PROBLEM DEFINITION

Having a shared understanding of the problem to address systems changes requires leadership. Leadership in facilitating systems change is not about one's position or who is at the top of the hierarchy. Leadership is something we all possess and can practice in any position in an organization. The role of systems leadership in defining adaptive, complex challenges is to encourage problem definition before solutions are proposed, to slow down—if even for a short while—to facilitate groups of people to jointly discuss, inquire, and define the problem rather than assume what it is and how it operates. Systems leaders also facilitate diverse participation and acknowledge and address power. Finally, systems leadership fosters the development of a vision for the future through collaborative learning and helps mobilize teams for action and growth.

Leading From the Middle, Leading From Anywhere as a Process of Systems Change

Traditional definitions of leadership assume that leadership is about who is in charge or has the most impressive title and includes only those people in positions of the highest authority. In contrast, a systems leader can lead from any position. Leadership is defined as a process that involves the facilitation of the active contribution of the skills of all people at all levels. Leading systems change in problem definition is about facilitating diverse groups to work collaboratively for the health of the whole system, rather than just pursuing quick, symptomatic fixes, and to develop pathways to address it that are not evident to any of us individually. It is a mindset, a set of skills and abilities, and the capacity to bring people together to ask questions and co-create a common future.

Facilitate Inquiry and Dialogue to Understand the Problem

One of the most crucial skill sets in problem definition is for leaders to help slow down the problem-solving process to explore the root causes that define systems challenges. Our fast-paced world demands quick decision-making and problem-solving. Systems challenges, however, cannot be solved quickly, and it is hard to solve a problem well (if at all) when we ignore its causes. Taking the time to define challenges often reveals that people have different perspectives of a problem; identify many different root causes, connections, and pathways; and see the situation from different levels in systems. Leaders need to have strong facilitation skills and ask questions to uncover the root of the issue and embrace different perspectives on why it is happening. Indeed, as Vogt et al. (2003) articulate in *The Art of Powerful Questions: Catalyzing Insight, Innovation and Action*:

> *As we enter an era in which systemic issues often lie at the root of critical challenges, in which diverse perspectives are required for sustainable solutions, and in which cause-and-effect relationships are not immediately apparent, the capacity to raise penetrating questions that challenge current operating assumptions will be key to creating positive futures.*[3(pp2–3)]

Promote Diverse Perspectives, Acknowledge Positionality, and Elevate Lived Experience

Systems leaders need to also ensure that all voices are heard to promote diversity, inclusion, and equity. These discussions often lead to new ideas and possibilities for addressing the situation. Leaders for systems change, as noted earlier, must possess robust facilitation skills and draw on these skills in framing discussion, dialogue, and inquiry. Leaders should help participants realize their positionality (i.e., one's power in culturally shaped structures of privilege and in organizational hierarchies, historically and now) and ensure that all people have a voice, no matter their background and experience. Individuals of color and with lived experience of inequity should be acknowledged and heard. In today's polarized civic society, especially in the United States, there are increasing calls for exploring divergences through open-ended dialogue before becoming invested in coming up with solutions, which requires a different frame for discussion.

Promote Vision Development and Collaborative Learning

Leadership for systems change is also about vision. Understanding the problem enables us to see opportunities. As Senge et al. say, leadership in systems thinking "helps people move beyond just reacting to these problems to building positive visions for the future."[4(p29)] Leaders who foster collective reflection and more generative conversations can help facilitate co-creation and co-design of the vision. This shared understanding of the future and the pathways forward promotes transformative learning, which helps us to think and act in new ways that reshape the system.

APPROACHES TO PROBLEM DEFINITION

To understand complex problems more deeply, we use systems science. Systems science or systems theory is an interdisciplinary field that is conceptually grounded in a concern with "interrelationships between parts and their relationships to a functioning whole."[5(p515)] There are several approaches or methodologies for systems science/theory used in public health, including soft-systems methodology, system dynamics, agent-based modeling, and network analysis. Each of these approaches has a role in problem definition; Table 9.1 defines each type of approach and its role in problem definition, and provides an example.

To understand problem definition, we primarily use soft-systems methodology. Soft-systems methodology was created by systems thinkers, including Peter Checkland, Brian Wilson, and Gerald Midgley[6,7] and Bob Williams.[8] Soft-systems approaches facilitate seeing the connections among perspectives, drawing boundaries, and identifying key interrelationships. In general, this is true of all systems approaches that facilitate discussion and analysis of alternative perceptions of a system to be considered. However, soft-systems methodology

TABLE 9.1 Definitions of Systems Science to Define Public Health Problems

EXAMPLES OF SYSTEMS SCIENCE METHODS	DEFINITION	USE IN PUBLIC HEALTH PROBLEM DEFINITION OR ASSESSMENT
Soft-Systems Methodology (SSM)	A problem-structuring approach when the problem definition is not apparent. Usually a qualitative, people-focused approach. SSM includes approaches to systems analysis that are less positivistic and "hard science," emphasizing the role of the observer of a system in constituting the system and contributing to the intractability or solubility of a problem.	SSM includes tools and techniques for generating alternative descriptions of a problem and discovering useful ways of reframing the problem.
System Dynamics (SD)	Structured approach for developing and testing mechanistic models of system behavior (i.e., how system structure produces observed, hoped for, or feared outcomes over time). Notable for its endogenous perspective, which encourages modelers to broaden their perspective and ask how system responses might reinforce and/or counteract earlier changes.	SD includes tools for qualitative modeling and aggregate or population-based computer simulation analyzing feedback links and loops and discovering leverage points. Running simulation models with different values of parameters helps us to understand the possibilities for the behavior of a system.

(*continued*)

TABLE 9.1 Definitions of Systems Science to Define Public Health Problems (*continued*)

EXAMPLES OF SYSTEMS SCIENCE METHODS	DEFINITION	USE IN PUBLIC HEALTH PROBLEM DEFINITION OR ASSESSMENT
Agent-Based Modeling	Uses computational models for simulating action and interactions of autonomous agents (individual or collective) to then assess the impacts on the system as a whole, e.g., income and food store type. "Hybrid" models can include both individual- and aggregate- (population) level actions.	Agent-based modeling helps us understand emergent phenomena that cross-cut ecological levels: how individual behavior can result in shifts in how a system behaves at an aggregate or population level. This modeling can inform and test plans for intervention.
Network Analysis	Focuses on relationships among entities within a system—between individual people, organizations, places, or jobs. Create quantitative measures of the degree and types of interconnections of entities within a system.	Explore contacts for communicable disease control, or alternatively model inter organizational relationships, for example, in PSE-related coalitions.

approaches focus more on the human definition and perception of problematic situations and the interrelationships of their components, and on how discussion of this in dialogue with others can promote learning. Promoting collaborative learning is vital to creating and leading systems change as each person becomes open to alternative problem definitions and pathways to address them, pilots the new pathway, and reflects on what worked and what did not, thereby facilitating learning. Exhibit 9.1 describes key considerations for perspectives, boundaries, and interrelationships.

A PROCESS TO UNDERSTAND ROOT CAUSES AND PROBLEM DEFINITION TO ADDRESS SYSTEMS CHANGE

While there is no one way to understand the root causes and define a problem to address systems change, we propose a six-step collective group process based on systems science concepts and our experiences (Exhibit 9.2). Before we share the comprehensive approach, we have a few caveats. First, this process is presented linearly; however, problem definition for complex problems usually requires cycling through these steps multiple times. Second, tools proposed in this chapter are meant to be a sampling of useful tools; others can be

EXHIBIT 9.1 Key Considerations for Perspectives, Boundaries, and Interrelationships

1. **Perspectives: Surface multiple points of view**
   a. Allow all voices to be heard from all walks of life and experience.
   b. Articulate assumptions explicitly.
   c. Foster engagement in co-creation and shared design of initiatives or interventions.
   d. Discuss ethical and power dynamics.
2. **Boundaries: Question what boundaries have been drawn and why**
   a. Ask what boundaries have been drawn and who is drawing them. "Boundaries" include how we delimit and define the categories, units, and concepts that are relevant to our problem or situation. If we are seeing, for example, the stigma of seeking mental health in our community as a problem, how is "mental health" defined and who is defining it; who is a member of our community, who is determining that, and what are the consequences of seeking services; how are we defining "stigma," what is it we are trying to reduce, and would others define it the same way? Another boundary we draw is the timeframe we choose when studying a problem—are we looking only at short term dynamics, or the long-term (e.g., life course or inter generational) effects?
   b. Facilitate discussion around the scope of the situation—are we considering partners at various levels (e.g., local, regional, state, national) and sectors (e.g., health, public safety, industry, education)?
   c. Within a set of boundaries/scope, appreciate and foster interconnections.
3. **Interrelationships**
   a. Look for circles of causality (feedback loops), which can be even more powerful drivers of change over time than linear causation. These include reinforcing and balancing loops. Reinforcing loops are often referred to as "vicious cycles" or "virtuous cycles." For example, less exercise leads to de-conditioning and greater difficulty in exercising, which leads to less exercising, or, once exercise is at the level to produce endorphins, more exercise leads to more desire to exercise, which leads to more exercise. Balancing loops counteract earlier changes, seeking balance or preventing "runaway" behavior, for example, a species' population growth exhausts food sources resulting in starvation that moderates the exponential, self-reinforcing population growth.
   b. Identify persistent patterns underlying dynamically complex situations (not just surface conditions or behaviors).
   c. Explore alternate connections and opportunities.

integrated as needed. Lastly, because we may not be able to take the time to deeply understand a problem and a resolution is needed quickly, we recommend a rapid-cycle problem definition process: (a) gather a few diverse perspectives on the challenge—dialogue or reflect ways to define the problem; (b) explore a few other examples of approaches to moving forward; and (c) map out implications before finalizing the solutions.

In the following, we define each step, its purpose, and associated tools or processes that can help accomplish its goal. The steps are outlined in Exhibit 9.2. Table 9.2 crosswalks the step, its purpose, and tools that can help complete the process.

Step 1: Getting Started: Develop a Team and Set Ground Rules With a "Not-Knowing" Mindset

First, a healthy team is a critical component of leading systems change. When we first begin to understand a complex problem, typically we start with a small group internal to our organization or partners within an ongoing collaboration. Ideally, your team should include individuals with different positions and perspectives from different levels within an organizational structure—the more diverse the better; this will likely uncover a broader understanding and more opportunities to address the problem. As we cycle through several versions of the steps, we are likely to expand the diversity and include more stakeholders outside of our initial group. Second, the team should set ground rules or participation principles that encourage diverse discussion and strong facilitation. Third, establish as a part of these ground rules a "not-knowing" open and growth mindset that encourages asking questions. Finally, set up a process to reflect and promote learning. Be sure to pause between each of the steps to reflect on what new information was gathered and how it added or changed the group's thinking and what new questions are now underway. This is important to ensure the group is on the same page; it also helps practice a growth mindset. Leading systems change is about embracing this step to ensure the team is ready to begin the process.

EXHIBIT 9.2 Steps to Understand the Root Cause and Define a Problem to Address Systems Change

- Step 1: Getting started: Develop a team and set ground rules with a "not-knowing" mindset.
- Step 2: Define the starting point for understanding the "situation of interest" and identify missing perspectives.
- Step 3: Describe multiple ways of defining a system from the points of view of those who have different perspectives about the system.
- Step 4: Organize the information and create themes.
- Step 5: Interpret the information to explore options for systems change.
- Step 6: Develop a vision and a theory of change (ToC) to guide work and process for ongoing individual and shared learning.
- Ongoing: Foster shared learning throughout the process.

TABLE 9.2 Crosswalk of Root Cause and Problem Definition Steps, Definitions, and Tools

STEPS TO DEFINING THE PROBLEM	WHAT IS PURPOSE OF THIS STEP?	WHAT ARE TOOLS TO HELP ACCOMPLISH THE STEP?
Step 1: Develop a team, set ground rules with a "not-knowing" mindset	Prepare a team with diverse representatives, set ground rules for engagement, and agree on a "not-knowing" mindset	See Chapter 7 on teams and cross-sector leadership
Step 2: Define the starting point for understanding the situation of interest and identify missing perspectives	Develop a starting point to inquire about the "situation of interest"	Reflective writing exercise The Public Health Learning Agenda Toolkit The five Rs framework
Step 3: Describe multiple mental models and ways of defining a system from different perspectives (or from different points of view) involved in the situation	Gather diverse perspectives about the situation of interest to capture others' understanding and approaches to addressing the situation	Informal interviewing Storytelling Rich pictures
Step 4: Organize the information and create themes	Organize the information into themes and understand where there are points of convergence or divergence	Card sort(ing) Mind-mapping
Step 5: Interpret the information to explore options for systems change	Interpret the perspectives based on stakeholders' role, positionality, power, and resources in the systems to help understand options for proceeding	Frames and stakes BATWOVE
Step 6: Develop a vision and a theory of change to guide your ongoing learning	Define the final outcome, your vision, and the approaches to exploring how to accomplish your work	Theory of change
Ongoing: Foster continuous learning	Reflect on where the team started, what was learned, and what new questions have emerged at each step of the process to promote shared learning	O.R.I.D.

Step 2: Define the Starting Point for Understanding the Situation of Interest and Identify Missing Perspectives

First, start by articulating the problem or situation of interest to explore. We recommend referring to a "situation of interest" at this step rather than "problem" because we don't want group members to assume there is a problem, what it is, or how it looks. One person may define the situation of interest as a problem while another does not. Further, the group has not yet defined the system and its scope yet. Using terminology like "situation of interest" can help group members avoid solidifying assumptions about "the problem" too early.

Defining a starting point for understanding the situation of interest can be overwhelming. How do we begin to learn more about inequities in maternal mortality, for example? One way to begin is to ask each team member to articulate, in writing, a description of the situation. Ask yourselves the questions listed in Exhibit 9.3.

The Public Health Learning Agenda Toolkit

Next, we want to ensure that we don't rush to a technical solution too soon. If anyone feels an adaptive solution is needed, we need to listen, given our tendency to "lean on" our expertise and evidence in technical ways. To do this, we want to share our perspectives with each team member and look for what is similar and what is different. Challenge each other as to whether what is shared is a technical or adaptive challenge, and whether the level of impact desired goes beyond a simple solution. One tool to help understand this is the Public Health Learning Agenda Toolkit,[9] available at www.publichealthlearningagenda.org. This toolkit takes us through key questions and provides tools we can use to facilitate discussion about whether a challenge is technical or adaptive and at what systems level we are trying to create change (Tool 1). Tool 1 asks critical but basic questions to help the team decide the type and depth of the problem.

EXHIBIT 9.3 Questions to Reflect and Write About When Defining a Starting Point

1. What is "the problem" as you see it? How would you describe it as a "situation of interest"?
2. What assumptions might you be making about what "the problem" is that could be limiting your solutions to the problem (e.g., is it a problem of inadequate education and knowledge conferral to pregnant women or a problem that access to choices and resources is lacking)?
3. What are examples of how people perceive "the problem" and how it occurs?
4. What is your understanding of why this problem exists? What are possible root or underlying causes? What do others think is the cause of the "the problem"?
5. Describe your future desire for what might happen if "the problem" is solved. Describe what you know about others' desires for an improved future state.

It presents a picture of the systems levels through an iceberg—whereby the technical challenges with more obvious solutions are at the top of the iceberg visible to all and the complex challenges with less obvious solutions are underneath the water. Once you have defined your challenge, the Public Health Learning Agenda Toolkit can also help you develop a plan to promote training and learning for systems change.

The Five Rs Framework

One process that can help define the "situation of interest" and help people understand others' perspectives on the problem is a framework called the five Rs. The five Rs framework was introduced as one of several system-mapping strategies to strengthen local systems at the U.S. Agency for International Development (USAID).[10] It's a simple set of questions that can lead to rich conversation. The five Rs include a series of questions focused on Results, Roles, Rules, Resources, and Relationships. These questions are provided in Exhibit 9.4; when addressed, they produce rich insights for any problem-solving initiative. The first R, Results, helps narrow the boundary, or focus of work. Looking at Results begins the process to identify shared measures of success. The second R, Roles, provides the opportunity to revisit and broaden a team, ensuring all stakeholders with a potential role in affecting (or who are affected by) change in prioritized Results are engaged. Discussion of the last three Rs—Rules, Resources, and Relationships—help us understand the system in which we're working. Rules shape Results and need to be worked with or changed. We don't want to fail to leverage available Resources (or address gaps). Critical Relationships need to be centered in change efforts. Given the adaptive nature of many public health problems and our efforts to strengthen systems, updating the five Rs over time can guide iterations to our approach, or allow us to follow up on problems we must address.

There are many options for brainstorming using the five Rs. Asynchronously, you can conduct a survey followed by group discussion of synthesized results or collect and organize responses through document sharing. Synchronous brainstorming sessions can be facilitated using nominal group techniques (sharing ideas, one at a time, around the room) while team members cluster responses to identify themes. The objective of this process is to brainstorm question responses, identify themes, fill in the gaps with additional brainstorming/interviewing, and then debrief the process and findings with the whole team. We recommend retaining as much of individuals' language as possible when grouping responses into themes. Doing so transparently can support individuals feeling heard and the development of a common vocabulary.

For more information about applying the five Rs to your process, explore the five Rs framework in the Program Cycle from USAID.[11]

Step 3: Gather Diverse Perspectives and Explore the Situation of Interest

Understanding the problem requires us to gather different stakeholders and organizations to broaden the definition of and opportunities for addressing the challenge at

EXHIBIT 9.4 The Five Rs Framework Questions

* Results: What does success look like? Start broadly, and then identify results everyone can get behind.
* Roles: Who has a role in effecting these results? Who is affected by change? (These are our key stakeholders, and we want to make sure to bring each key stakeholder into this and subsequent conversations.)
* Resources: What do we have, not just money or grants, but assets and other strengths, to create change?
* Rules: What are the formal (e.g., regulations, laws, eligibility requirements) and informal rules (e.g., norms, culture) that affect how things work? We need to design change initiatives with these in mind, changing them sometimes and working within these constraints at other times.
* Relationships: What are the most important relationships we need to be aware of in making change? Relationships connect two nouns—people, organizations, characteristics of the environment, or tasks. Call out what matters most in getting to key results.

hand. This step includes collecting diverse perspectives from people outside our current team, ideally from completely different sectors than you've worked with before and public documents and websites, if applicable. The goal is to understand others' interpretation, definition of "the problem" and its causes, and what they may already be doing to address it. Additionally, try to understand how these partners do their work, including how they are organized. What is their organizational system? Often, other stakeholders have already considered the problem and worked to address it, or they have skills or strengths that we can learn from.

To get started, we need to be clear about the most current definition of the problem our team agreed upon since it likely went through several iterations after applying the five Rs framework. We also need to clarify the questions we want to answer and how we will collect information in a standard way. Next, we want to compare our own perceptions of "the problem." An emphasis should be made on helping our team and stakeholders tell their lived experiences—what has happened and how problems are being experienced at the community level. There are several ways to gather diverse stakeholder information. Two strategies include storytelling and creating rich pictures, described in the next sections.

Storytelling

Storytelling can be an effective way to elicit and compare different perspectives on a problem or situation from a personal point of view. To practice storytelling, start by getting specific descriptions of how events and activities relevant to the "situation of interest" have unfolded, from the perspectives of the multiple stakeholders involved. The lead facilitator should ask the team or stakeholders to tell their stories about their experience with the issue of interest. Always start with the stakeholder's concrete experience as told through a story. Do not begin by being too analytical and asking a stakeholder to define the problem, but probe for the stakeholder to describe a time when the person experienced the "situation of interest"—what happened, what went well, what did not, why might this have happened, and so forth. Hearing details of stakeholders' lived experiences of the "situation of interest" will facilitate a more descriptive, authentic, and deeper description with their stories. This approach also helps to address any power dynamic that may exist between you and the stakeholder by removing the likelihood that the stakeholder will share only what they think you want to hear.

Rich Pictures

Another way of getting people to communicate their lived experience about a "situation of interest" and what they see as problematic (or not) about it is to draw the concrete elements and relationships involved on a large sheet of paper. This can be done in a group to surface multiple perspectives, using the drawings to start conversations about what is seen and experienced from diverse positions. "Rich pictures" should be messy—they are a visual way to support a "brain dump"—a way for people to externalize without too much censoring the multiple actors, aspects of the contexts, feelings (via smiley or frowny faces, jagged lines, etc.) that they see as pertinent to the situation—that's what makes them "rich." People should be encouraged to draw images—they can also include key words and phrases—that are evocative of what they have seen and felt. They can use connecting curves and arrows to show connections and relationships. Arrows and lines should be labeled so you as the viewer can understand the drawer's intention as opposed to reading into what you think should be there. The value of the pictures lies in the conversations that can be catalyzed; be sure to allow time for discussion and debriefing. For more information about how to ask partners to draw rich pictures, visit The Better Evaluation website at www .betterevaluation.org.[12]

Step 4: Organize the Information and Create Themes

We have collected a lot of great information. How do we organize it in meaningful ways? How do we examine the different perspectives to make sense of who said what? We want to understand what people said that was similar but also what was said that was unique or different. The goal of this step is to walk away with clear statements that your team can agree on about what your information currently says and determine if there are themes aligned with specific perspectives or people in different positions (i.e., who may or may not have more power than others). This will help prepare the team for Step 5. Two strategies to organize your information meaningfully are card sort and mind-mapping.

Card Sort(ing)

Card sorting is a clustering strategy to help a team make meaning of what has been shared through the strategies outlined in Steps 1 through 4. When sharing perspectives and brainstorming, it is important to hear from diverse perspectives—explaining things in individuals' own words, based on their own mental models. It is important to keep this detailed "divergent" information. But organizing information and making sense of it requires "convergent" thinking. Card sorting is a tool to assist with sense making. With card sorting, you write individual words/phrases about meaningful results or key root causes of a problem, for example, on individual sticky notes or index cards that can be sorted into groups. You can even include elements from rich pictures. Each group is then named to identify emergent themes. This can also be done electronically by moving text within a document or table. Identified themes can be summarized to enhance a growing understanding of the situation of interest. Because analysts' perspectives affect interpretation, it is important that clustering be transparent and not done by any individual alone. Results of clustering can be used to spur more divergent thinking about what is missing, allowing the cycle to continue until saturation is reached—that is, participants are satisfied with all key themes that have surfaced. As situations evolve, understanding may change and this process of linking more specific ideas to themes can support such iterative updating.

Mind-Mapping

Another way to help sort information is through a process called mind-mapping. Mind-mapping helps teams diagram stakeholder information and feedback information in a visual way, organizing the information by themes, words, activities, or other concepts, linking or arranging the information around a core concept in a non linear way. There are six easy steps to creating a mind map. You can either draw out your mind map on a piece of paper or computer, or there is free mind-mapping software you can use. The basic steps include: (a) define the problem you are focused on at the center of the map; (b) brainstorm or use the topics that are related to the problem to create "branches" connected to the center; (c) create any subtopics connected to the branches; and (d) discuss the arrangement and organization of the themes and what they mean. These steps and more instructions are described in detail on the Mind-Mapping website at www.mindmapping .com.[13]

Step 5: Analyze and Interpret the Information

Once you have organized the information in a way that people can easily review, it is time to interpret and decide what it means. We know that perspectives are often seemingly weighted by people's roles and power in the system. It is important for systems change that we explore these roles carefully and see how these points of view might change our decisions around what first steps we take toward learning and action. There are several systems tools that help us with this analysis. Ultimately, the group will need to decide which definition of the problem and its causes resonates with multiple stakeholders relevant to your organization, community, and/or systems needs and assets. Two specific tools include: frames and stakes and BATWOVE. These tools are described in the following.

Frames and Stakes

For a clear roadmap for collecting information about frames and stakes, and surfacing and critiquing assumptions about "the problem," who has a stake in it, and what stake(s) they have, see Bob Williams's workbook, *Wicked Solutions.*[8] If this tool is applied after five Rs, rich pictures, and storytelling, we should have a list of stakeholders in the situation of interest or problem. We can then discuss this list in a group that includes people with different perspectives and sources of information to see if anyone has been left out. If so, we may decide to return to earlier steps to collect additional stakeholder input.

For each stakeholder, discuss the extent of their involvement in the situation and what stake they have in it. For key (i.e., greatly involved) stakeholders, the group can discuss what their stake in "the situation/problem" is: what their relevant goals are, what they are seeking from potential outcomes, how it benefits them, and what they value. Allow for disagreement and for discussion to change your own and the group's understandings of possible stakes. Then consider how these stakes relate to different ways of framing the problem or situation. See if the group can collectively come up with at least three different ways of framing the problem. For example, is the problem about reducing disease as much as possible? About balancing risks and benefits of being open versus closed so as to benefit kids as much as possible? Or about deciding about being open or closed based on the objective of maximizing equity in outcomes during the pandemic?

Different stakeholders and stakes result in different understandings of what "the problem" is, ways of drawing the boundaries around a system of interest, and defining the key relationships. Once we have surfaced alternative ways of framing "the problem," then we can discuss as a group the most useful way of defining "the problem" and what will resonate with key stakeholders. Then we can support a pathway to move forward including, if appropriate, a plan for intervention.

BATWOVE

BATWOVE is a soft-systems acronym that built on the earlier soft-systems CAT-WOE questions (clients or customers, actors/agents, transformation statement, worldview, owner, environment).[14] BATWOVE as a tool includes discussing and defining: (a) T—a transformation statement, (b) A—agents or actors, (c) B—beneficiaries or victims, (d) O—owners, (e) W—worldview, and (f) E—environment. ("BATWOVE" is a pronounceable way to remember the elements, but the order of the letters does not reflect directions for the order in which to discuss them.) Each of these elements is described in the following with suggested questions to support definition and discussion. The transformation statement is listed first, but we may wish to discuss the other elements before discussing and articulating the transformation statement, or begin with it and then come back to it. Discussing the transformation statement and the other elements results in summarizing and clarifying the group's understanding of a problem/situation of interest and their proposed plan to deal with it (the transformation statement).

Transformation statement: This is a capsule plan for an intervention and is a one-sentence theory of change (ToC), in the form "do P (what), by Q (how), to achieve R (why)." You can ask, "What do we think we want to do? How are we going to do this—what specific methods and activities are we planning? Why are we planning to do this—what do we want to achieve?" For instance, "[what] Help pregnant women get resources they need to stay healthy during pregnancy, [how] by training and supporting a cadre of community health workers who will provide counseling and coaching to pregnant women in X and Y communities, [why] because counseling and coaching is known to have the greatest impact on birth outcomes when it is provided by someone relateable and with whom a sustained relationship—and thus sustained coaching—is more likely to happen." The template for transformation statements can be a useful tool in involving a group of stakeholders to discuss what will become the parameters of a ToC. Transformation statements should be developed and brought into thorough dialogue among a stakeholder group after different possibilities for framing the problem and solutions are discussed.

Actors/agents: Ask, "Who is taking actions that affect this situation? Think of people, but also organizations or other groups of people who collectively act or make decisions." Actors or agents are the key people or organizations whose actions are relevant to "the problem" as currently defined.

B and V (Beneficiaries and victims): Once we have come up with a potential idea for intervention, or "transformation," ask, "Who are the potential beneficiaries and victims?" People (especially in the governmental or nonprofit sectors) are often resistant to talking about victims, but this is important in creating practical solutions. For instance, maybe there are some people in our organizations who act as gatekeepers to particular procedures or processes that would be changed by the proposed intervention, and maybe they feel that these changes threaten their roles and/or jobs. For the intervention to be successful, this is something we need to address.

"Owners": Ask, "Who are the 'owners'—who controls this situation? Who could stop a proposed change from going forward?" Owners have a different level of control over the situation than other actors. They aren't merely taking relevant actions, but their action or inaction can halt a proposed intervention.

"Worldview": Ask the group, "What are the worldviews that are reflected in the actions of the actors/agents in this situation we are describing? That is, what assumptions are they making about what outcomes are important and valuable, or to be avoided? What stake or 'skin in the game' do they have in outcomes from this situation, and how does that affect how they act and react? Are there ways in which divergent worldviews from different actors are affecting the situation?" Worldview refers to the perspectives that are described when we probe for the "stakes" or "skin in the game" perceived by

actors in the system. Beyond immediate benefit or lack thereof, inquiring about world-view includes inquiring about stakeholders' underlying values. They may or may not articulate these explicitly; sometimes they have to be inferred from action or from the way that stakeholders tell stories about their involvement. Understanding where worldviews may be divergent versus convergent is frequently important in public settings and important to address when considering implications for equity.

Define "environment": Ask, "What aspects of the environment—social, political, economic, physical—are affecting the situation we are discussing?" All these contexts surrounding the problem or situation are important to consider in planning and successfully implementing a proposed transformation or intervention.

All these questions clarifying the elements in "BATWOVE" should be discussed in a diverse stakeholder group and not just analyzed in isolation by public health experts. This discussion creates a shared understanding that is a foundation for collectively moving forward to intervention.

Step 6: Set a Vision and a Theory of Change: What Are We Going to Do Now?

Based on the information collected and synthesized through the previous steps, the group should develop a shared definition of the problem, articulate a vision for the future, and outline how it wants to reach that vision. In this crucial step, the team should keep in mind group values and team principles so that no one voice outweighs any other in the decision process. It is also important to keep in mind that there does not need to be a final decision or answer; rather, iterative cycles of piloting, testing, and improving the team's capacity may be needed to begin to address the problem. More work may need to be completed to clarify the problem, repeating the process described.

To get started with moving toward a problem definition, vision, and approach to taking action, a ToC is useful. ToC is a commonly used approach for diverse groups of stakeholders to collectively map out the logical sequence of changes with their contextual conditions to support the desired long-term change for complex public health challenges.[15] ToC uses our data and information and articulated assumptions about what we think is really going on to help set an outcome or vision, identify a feasible pathway forward, including stepping-stones or activities or interventions that will realistically help us get there. Eventually, the result is a roadmap, including a strategy agenda with goals and action plans and an evaluation and measurement tool with associated process, impact, and outcome metrics.

There are many resources for learning about ToC[16] (e.g., TheoryofChange.org).

Adapting ToC approaches from our past experiences, we propose a four-step process. Step 1 involves defining the ultimate outcome and related challenges. Using data and information you've collected about the situation of interest (e.g., results in Five Rs), identify the biggest challenge at hand—what the ultimate outcome is that your team should resolve. Then identify 3 to 5 challenges that relate to this ultimate outcome; these are intermediate outcomes. The desired ultimate outcome should project the success of your work and serve as a vision. Step 2 defines what must happen to address the challenges you've identified. Ask yourself, what has to happen in order for these intermediate and, thus, the ultimate outcomes to occur? What programs, efforts, or activities are happening now, and how do they relate to your outcomes? What new approaches may be needed? Select the activities, programs, or initiatives ("interventions") that align best with how you think you can address your challenges/intermediate outcomes of interest. Step 3 creates connections and pathways between the ultimate outcome, intermediate outcomes, and interventions needed for these to occur. As you make these connections, ask yourself what assumptions you are making about these connections. Is there a certain way in which you are doing your work, for example, focusing on individual change versus population-level change? These assumptions inform your overall strategies for the ToC. Finally, in Step 4 you should document how you will evaluate your success; how will you assess what you have learned and document what needs to be adapted along the way? While part of the ToC pushes you to think about interventions and measures—perhaps earlier than your team might feel ready—your early thinking will help you more clearly articulate the root challenge your team is striving to address. In articulating interventions and measures of success, stakeholders will disclose their mental models more fully about what root challenges matter most in creating change. As the project evolves, you should be sure to go back and update your ToC.

Ongoing: Set Up a Learning Process

As the team begins and between each step, set up a process for reflection and learning. It is important to build trust and ensure the team members are on the same page by taking time to reflect on where we were, where we are, what was learned, and where we might be going. One tool that can help with this reflection is the Institute for Cultural Affairs Technology of Participation facilitation approach called the Art of the Focused Conversation. One core component to this approach is the facilitation technique of O.R.I.D.[17] The O.R.I.D. framework promotes reflection of shared information or experiences and helps participants see different points of view, reflect on the meaning of the situation, and determine next steps. The basic framework is shown in Exhibit 9.5.

EXHIBIT 9.5 O.R.I.D. Framework

O: Objective questions about what "data" each person experienced or took away
R: Reflective questions on how the experience or information made each
    person feel or how they reacted
I: Interpretative questions about what the information or experience might
    mean to the person, group, or situation overall
D: Decisional questions that elicit what learning occurred, what new questions
    arose, or what can be done next to move forward

CHAPTER SUMMARY

Defining "the problem" or challenge is a crucial beginning step to lead systems change. However, rushing that process and assuming that everyone agrees on the problem definition, and then jumping ahead to a solution, can lead to ineffective and inefficient results. Systems challenges are complex because often there are many perspectives in how the challenge is defined. Surfacing these multiple perspectives is necessary to promote the mutual learning and deep understanding of root causes and drivers needed to achieve enduring, transformative change. Without a deeper analysis of the root causes to the problem, we are in danger of continuing to address only surface-level challenges that are downstream and technical, rather than addressing the adaptive issues of structural and social determinants of health. Systems leaders need to facilitate conversations that ask questions and promote critical thinking, welcome diverse perspectives that support creativity and innovation, and allow the time and deliberation necessary to integrate those perspectives into a collective vision of the future. This chapter outlines a framework with a step-by-step process and exercises that public health leaders can use to discuss and define problems from a systems perspective and begin to take action while co-learning with partners along the way.

Key Messages

1. Complex problems are difficult because people often have different world views about our environment. Defining the systems depends on our perspective, and power and positionality can impact the process.
2. Leading systems change is about having mindset, a set of skills and abilities, and the capacity to bring people together to ask questions and co-create toward a common future, regardless of one's position in an organization or system. Leaders facilitate inquiry and dialogue to understand the problem; promote diverse perspectives, acknowledge positionality, and elevate lived experience; and promote vision development and collaborative learning.
3. There are many types of systems science that can be used for problem definition. This chapter focuses on soft-systems methodology, which emphasizes the importance of dialogue and learning to understand perspectives, boundaries, and interrelationships.
4. While there is no one or right way, we propose a six-step approach to problem definition to help identify root causes and reveal possible generative pathways forward to address the challenge at hand. This chapter outlines a process and exercises that can help to define problems from a systems perspective and begin to act while learning along the way.

Tips

1. As a systems leader, resist the temptation to jump to action or a solution without clarifying a definition of the problem or "situation" of interest. Instead, facilitate diverse perspectives to help understand the situation and co-create a vision for the future.
2. If you are short on time, consider a rapid-cycle problem definition process to have a basic understanding of where you are starting from: (a) gather a few diverse perspectives on the challenge—dialogue or reflect ways to define the problem; (b) explore a few other examples of approaches to moving forward; and (c) map out implications before finalizing the solutions.
3. Start this process with a "not-knowing" mindset to help remain open to different understandings of the situation, explore root causes and see the adaptive challenges, and novel pathways to address the problem at hand.

Supplemental Resources

- The Public Health Learning Agenda: https://publichealthlearningagenda.org/
- The 5Rs in 5 minutes: www.mchnavigator.org/transformation/systems-integration.php
- Get the Big Picture—Draw a Rich Picture: www.betterevaluation.org/en/resources/overview/get_the_big_picture
- Wicked Solutions—A Systems Approach to Complex Problems: www.lulu.com/shop/bob-williams-and-sjon-van-t-hof/wicked-solutions-a-systems-approach-to-complex-problems/paperback/product-22562407.html?page=1&pageSize=4
- The Community Builder's Approach to Theory of Change: www.mspguide.org/sites/default/files/resource/aspen_institute_-_the_community_builders_guide_to_theory_of_change.pdf
- Technology of Participation (ToP)—Facilitation Training: www.top-training.net/w/

REFERENCES

1. COVID-19 racial and ethnic health disparities. Centers for Disease Control and Prevention website. https://www.cdc.gov/coronavirus/2019-ncov/community/health-equity/racial-ethnic-disparities/index.html. Updated December 10, 2020. Accessed January 18, 2021.
2. Williams B, Hummelbrunner R. *Systems Concepts in Action: A Practitioner's Toolkit.* Stanford; 2011:17. Introduction.
3. Vogt E, Brown J, Isaacs D. *The Art of Powerful Questions: Catalyzing Insight, Innovation and Action.* Whole Systems Associates; 2003.
4. Senge P, Hamilton H, Kania J. The dawn of system leadership. *Stanf Soc Innov Rev.* 2015;13(1):27–33. doi:10.48558/YTE7-XT62.

5. Trochim WM, Cabrera DA, Milstein B, Gallagher RS, Leischow SJ. Practical challenges of systems thinking and modeling in public health. *Am J Public Health*. 2006;96(3):538–546, quote on page 539. Cited by: Frerichs L, Lich KH, Dave G, et al. Integrating systems science and community-based participatory research to achieve health equity. *Am J Public Health* 2016;106(2):215–222.
6. Checkland P. *Systems Thinking, Systems Practice*. Wiley; 1999.
7. Wilson B. *Soft Systems Methodology Conceptual Model Building and Its Contribution*. Wiley; 2001.
8. Williams B, van 't Hof S. *Wicked Solutions: A Systems Approach to Complex Problems*. Lulu. com; 2016.
9. Welter C, Davis S, Lloyd L, et al. *Creating a Learning Agenda: A Toolkit to Foster Organizational Learning for Today's Public Health Challenges*. Public Health Training Centers; 2020. https:// publichealthlearningagenda.org/
10. Local systems: A framework for supporting sustained development. U.S. Agency for International Development website. https://www.usaid.gov/policy/local-systems -framework. Published May 1, 2014. Accessed January 18, 2021.
11. U.S. Agency for International Development. *The 5Rs Framework in the Program Cycle*. U.S. Agency for International Development. https://usaidlearninglab.org/sites/default/files/ resource/files/5rs_techncial_note_ver_2_1_final.pdf. Published October 2016. Accessed January 18, 2021.
12. Rich Pictures. Better Evaluation website. https://www.betterevaluation.org/en/evaluation -options/richpictures. Updated July 7, 2020. Accessed January 18, 2021.
13. Mindmapping. https://www.mindmapping.com/. Accessed January 18, 2021.
14. BATWOVE. Innovation Food Systems Teaching and Learning. https://www.ifstal.ac.uk/ wp-content/uploads/2018/07/Handout-WS4.pdf. Published 2018. Accessed January 18, 2021.
15. Breuer E, Lee L, De Silva M, et al. Using theory of change to design and evaluate public health interventions: a systematic review. *Implement Sci*. 2015;11(1):63.
16. Theory of Change Community Center for Theory of Change website. https://www .theoryofchange.org. Accessed January 18, 2021.
17. Stanfield RB (ed.). *The Art of Focused Conversation: 100 Ways to Access Group Wisdom in the Workplace*. New Society Publishers; 2000.

10

Leveraging the Lessons of Implementation Science to Serve Systems Change

W. Oscar Fleming

CHAPTER OBJECTIVES

By the end of this chapter, the practitioner will be able to:

- Understand the interrelated factors that influence the implementation of successful systems change.
- Carefully appraise and select innovations that are well suited for your context.
- Leverage implementation support competencies in your system and build those that are lacking.
- Use evidence-based implementation frameworks and tools to plan, guide, and evaluate complex change.
- Foster an enabling environment for change through robust collaboration and active learning strategies.

INTRODUCTION

Systems change leaders have a dual challenge.[1] On the one hand, they must be able to envision and communicate a better future, a new system capable of fostering enhanced well-being for all. On the other hand, they must come to understand the current system and its strengths and weaknesses so that they can intervene effectively. And for any chance at broad and sustained impact, systems change leaders must do this work collaboratively and in the context of ongoing, unpredictable change in policy and in political and community contexts.

The coronavirus disease 2019 (COVID-19) global pandemic underlines both the importance and difficulty of protecting and improving public health. Health and well-being are products of complex systems in which some elements, such as health promotion campaigns, are planned and manageable, whereas other elements, such as new infectious agents, are unexpected and unpredictable. Health is also influenced by multiple systems, including transportation, the economy, education, and more. These systems interact and have a dynamic impact on the public's health, complicating efforts to improve health and well-being.

In response to this complexity, efforts to improve health have evolved. Narrowly focused efforts, such as specific evidence-based interventions and policies, certainly have a role to play. However, these interventions work best when part of a comprehensive and aligned package of changes working at the individual, family, community, organizational, and policy levels. As a systems change leader, you need skills and tools to collaboratively plan, deliver, and improve this multilevel package of changes over time and in an evolving context.

Senge et al.[1] describe the three core capabilities of systems leaders, including (a) an ability to see the system, (b) fostering reflective and generative conversations, and (c) shifting from reactive to co-creative problem-solving. This chapter explores how leaders like you can use implementation science to bring these capabilities to life through practice. Implementation science is the study and use of methods to promote the uptake and integration of innovations to improve population well-being equitably.[2-4] This chapter begins with a definition of implementation science and examination of its relevance to systems change. The chapter explores the importance of operationalizing systems change "interventions" and continually assessing the context to inform decision-making. Next, the chapter addresses the importance of fostering an enabling context, including the need for leadership from and continuous learning among diverse stakeholders. The chapter ends with a reflection on the road ahead, including recommendations to expand the scope and pace of public health improvement. Specific frameworks, relevant research, and other resources are described in each section and summarized at the end.

DEFINING IMPLEMENTATION SCIENCE

Implementation science includes the study *and* use of methods to promote the systematic uptake and effective use of evidence-based interventions and other innovations to improve population health and well-being.[2-4] The science emerged in response to the significant time lag between the development of evidence-based interventions and their widespread uptake in practice. In addition, both researchers and practitioners have voiced concern about poor quality of implementation once adopted.[5] In response, a variety of theories, models, and frameworks (hereafter called frameworks) have been developed to describe the factors that (a) influence implementation, (b) guide implementation, and (c) define and measure relevant outcomes.[6] In summary, implementation science provides public health practitioners with guidance on selecting, delivering, and improving innovation use to realize improved outcomes. Systems change leaders like you can use this science to guide change efforts and strengthen systems capacity to support innovative approaches and practices.

The Active Implementation Formula[7] (see Figure 10.1) depicts the critical domains of any change effort. These domains—*Effective Innovations, Effective Implementation,* and *Enabling Context*—are explored throughout this chapter. *Effective Innovations* refers to the approaches used to improve the health and well-being of a given population or community. These approaches are the "what," that is, the programs, policies, and practices (e.g., policy change to expand funding for maternal health services) we implement to improve public health outcomes. The evidence base for these approaches ranges from strong to promising to nonexistent.[8]

Effective Implementation encompasses the "how," that is, the methods used to identify, prepare for, and deliver these innovations. A variety of strategies, working at various levels (e.g., service delivery, organizational, policy) within a system, are typically needed to identify, address, and manage contextually relevant facilitators and barriers. Finally, the *Enabling Context* domain speaks to the environment surrounding ("where") and the people ("with whom") involved in the change effort. Continuous learning and co-creation with diverse systems stakeholders are critical in this domain.

The formula organizes a complex and multifaceted range of activities into a few buckets. The work within and across the buckets is iterative and you will find yourself working in each simultaneously. The purpose of the formula is not to oversimplify the complexity of systems change, but to provide systems change leaders with a way to frame the primary components of the work in the face of its inherent complexity. The formula

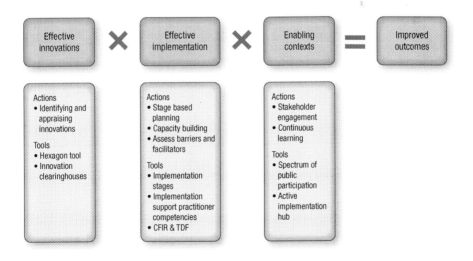

Figure 10.1 Active implementation formula.
Source: Reproduced with permission from Easterling D, Metz A. Getting real with strategy: insights from implementation science. *Foundation Rev.* 2016;8(2).
CFIR, Consolidated Framework for Implementation Research; TDF, Theoretical Domains Framework.

is used to organize this chapter and highlight six critical actions and relevant tools to support them (Figure 10.1). You can use the formula and these tools to understand and structure the many moving parts of a systems change effort, as described in the following.

EFFECTIVE INNOVATIONS AND SYSTEMS CHANGE

How Do I Identify and Select Effective Innovations?

One key and ongoing implementation task that you will face as a systems change leader is the selection of innovations to support prioritized changes. Innovations include policies (e.g., universal coverage for annual well-woman visits in health insurance plans), services (e.g., an adolescent health education program), and collaborative approaches (e.g., community based). You can identify these innovations and explore their purpose and related research through many available registries and databases.[9–11] In short, an innovation is what you implement to improve health outcomes.

Several collaborative methodologies have been developed to help diverse stakeholders come together to plan and support complex systems change. Examples of collaborative approaches you might consider include Collective Impact,[12] the PRO-moting School-community-university Partnerships to Enhance Resilience (PROSPER) model,[13] Results Based Accountability,[14] and Strategic Doing,[15] to name a few. In the following section, I explore how you can draw on the lessons of implementation science to guide the choice of a collaborative innovation.

Systems change innovations must be carefully selected to respond to the identified need and context. The work of identifying and selecting an innovation should be done by a group of invested stakeholders that represents the community and has the time and support to carefully consider multiple possible innovations. This "exploration team" should carefully appraise alternative innovations to determine their fit and feasibility in the context. This requires that the team develop a shared understanding of the context and a working knowledge of the core components of each innovation. For example, the Collective Impact approach defines five domains (e.g., common agenda, shared measurement, mutually reinforcing activities, continuous communication, backbone support) with linked substrategies that have been increasingly developed and operationalized.[12] Other models provide similar guidance and support, which is invaluable to teams during exploration.

Exploration teams must carefully review the evidence supporting the use of each innovation, including the evidence of efficacy and effectiveness as well as where and with whom the evidence was developed. While published research rarely provides adequate details, additional information can often be obtained from innovation developers, purveyors, and other technical assistance providers. Understanding the source of the evidence and the context of where it was developed can provide insights into its fit with the team's context. Considerations of the strength and sources of evidence can also be factored into later-stage plans for evaluation and continuous learning, as further discussed in the following.

The exploration team must also consider how usable the innovation will be in the context. Usability concerns the level of operationalization of the core components (i.e., detailed descriptions of how to carry them out). I often help teams consider the following questions: Are manuals and other resources available? Are there implementing sites that can share their experiences and lessons? The exploration team can identify supports available to help introduce the innovation into the context, including the purveyors and other technical assistance providers, as mentioned earlier. For example, the Collective Impact Forum supports learning collaboratives that help users learn from one another. The cost and scope of these supports are additional points to explore. The details gathered during a robust exploration process can guide subsequent efforts to translate the innovation to the local context during installation. What's more, this careful consideration of the innovation can identify areas for adaptation to improve fit with the context. Relevant tools to support such exploration efforts are presented in the following.

EFFECTIVE IMPLEMENTATION AND SYSTEMS CHANGE

The second element of the Active Implementation formula, Effective Implementation, concerns the evolving nature of implementation work and the methods used to facilitate change over time. The following section describes specific implementation frameworks you can use to strengthen the capacity to support successful systems change.

How Does Implementation Work Change Over Time?

Managing implementation in complex systems requires accounting for change over time. The Active Implementation Stages framework can help (Figure 10.2).[2,16] Stages (or phases) are a concept common to many implementation frameworks.[17,18] I use them throughout the chapter to ground the discussion in practical examples. As described earlier, during the *exploration* stage, you can work with teams to (a) assess population

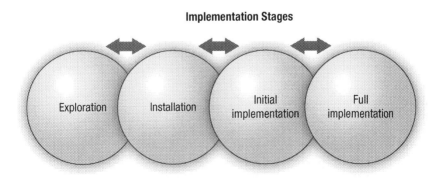

Figure 10.2 Implementation stages.
Source: Reproduced with permission from Fixsen D, Naoom SF, Blase KA, et al. *Implementation Research: A Synthesis of the Literature*. 1st ed. University of South Florida, Louis de la Parte Florida Mental Health Institute; 2005:1–125.

resources and needs, (b) define desired outcomes, and (c) select innovations. During the *installation* stage, your focus shifts to strengthening the infrastructure—the people, finances, material resources, processes, and relationships—needed for your chosen innovations. The work in this stage involves developing new partnerships, hiring staff, improving data systems, and much more.

Once you start using the innovation (e.g., your coalition is using a structured process to appraise different community-based approaches to improve maternal health in the community), you have moved into the *initial implementation* stage. Here, your focus evolves to include rapid assessment and quality improvement to identify and address the key factors influencing performance. You reach the final stage, *full implementation*, when you have achieved an established level of consistency, quality, and outcomes. For a service-focused innovation, this could be measured as consistent program fidelity among service providers. For a process-focused innovation like our coalition, this might be measured by meeting targets for membership diversity (of experience and representation), satisfaction, and productivity. For both types of innovations, ongoing improvement, capacity development, and thoughtful adaptation are key actions in this stage.

You can use a stage-based approach to integrate attention to sustainability from the very beginning. The stages help systems change leaders and collaborators make decisions about the work in front of them that is informed by the work to come. For example, in selecting a maternal health education campaign (exploration stage), you might help coalition partners to consider the potential to scale an innovation (full implementation stage) *if* it is found to be effective in the context. With this stage-based perspective, you can support more intentional, transparent, and early considerations of relevance, equity, cost, and feasibility.

I want to emphasize the following points in response to the complexity and scope of systems change. First, implementation is not linear. Installation activities (e.g., staff recruitment, training, coaching) often carry on throughout initial and full implementation. Furthermore, systems change efforts include multiple innovations that will be in different stages at the same time. I have supported county-level coalitions to improve their collaborative practices (initial implementation) while they simultaneously support the launch of a new home-visiting program (installation) and consider alternative approaches to improving early literacy (exploration). You don't need to use the stages to over simplify systems change, but rather to provide a useful way to plan, manage, and guide the work across the total portfolio.

How Can I Strengthen Systems Capacity to Support Change?

Once an innovation has been chosen, turn your attention to the workforce. As the nature and scope of the systems change effort emerges, change leaders must carefully reflect on the specific knowledge, skills, and abilities that will be needed to support and sustain the work. Key questions include:

- What critical competencies are needed?
- What level of capacity exists?

- What additional capacity is needed?
- How can partners and collaborators with the needed capacity be recruited?
- How can collaborators leverage their collective capacity for the larger good?
- What processes are needed to continually assess and strengthen our capacity?

To answer these questions, you must take the time to define and periodically assess the competencies and skill sets needed in the context. This will include innovation-specific competencies, as well as change facilitation competencies. Fortunately, emergent research has identified relevant competencies for leaders engaged in complex systems change implementation (Figure 10.3).[19] Six foundational principles (e.g., be curious) guiding how change leaders approach their work draw on decades of complex implementation research and practice. In addition, the three domains—co-creation and engagement, ongoing improvement, and sustaining change—organize a diverse range of specific competencies that are central to the complex work of change leadership. I encourage you to explore these in the context of your change effort.

I want to emphasize three points. First, the breadth of competencies corresponds to the complex nature of systems change. Because they are grounded in and draw on relevant research, you can work with your counterparts to assess and identify the capacity-building priorities in your context. Viable strategies can then be developed to address these priorities.

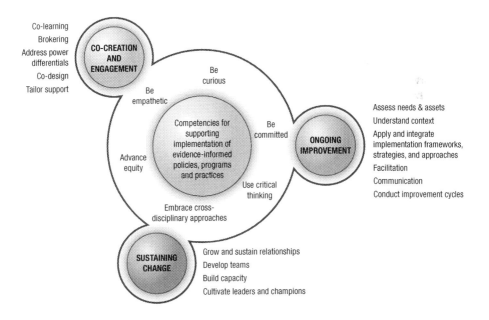

Figure 10.3 Principles and core competencies of implementation support practitioners.
Source: Reproduced with permission from Metz A, Burke K, Albers B, Louison L, Bartley L. *A Practice Guide to Supporting Implementation*. University of North Carolina at Chapel Hill, Chapel Hill, North Carolina. 2020.

Second, the breadth and scope of these competencies also highlight the inherent value of collective action. No single organization is likely to be able to develop and sustain this range of competencies. Fortunately, this is unnecessary. Instead, you can leverage your collaborative partnership to involve individuals with a mix of skills in the work.

Finally, it is unlikely that any individual will have or be able to develop skills in each competency area. This is also unnecessary. Instead, you can bring individuals with diverse skills together in teams to support specific aspects of the work. You can use available examples of structured, team-based approaches to inform your own approach.[20–22]

You likely already realize that recruitment and the development of the right mix of competencies among diverse collaborators is a key leadership role. While public health and other human service professionals may have relevant training and experience, many will not. Furthermore, community stakeholders will have valuable lived experience but may have less experience with formal collaborative processes. To develop the right mix of skills and perspectives, you will need sustained and committed effort supported by a subset of actors responsible for continually defining, assessing, and engaging the necessary actors.

You can use several strategies to strengthen the workforce. High-quality training has an important role to play but rarely leads to practice change on its own.[23] You will also need complementary approaches, including coaching and supportive supervision, which can support the translation of knowledge and skills gained from training into day-to-day practice. Next, you can develop and support learning processes that help collaborators use data to monitor progress and target improvement efforts. For example, a coalition could use the Wilder Collaborative Factors Inventory to periodically assess coalition functioning, using the findings to prioritize quality improvement efforts.[24] Depending on the culture and history of the partners within the system, you should carefully introduce, normalize, and transparently facilitate such learning strategies to overcome fear of retribution and blame that has often been a part of systems cultures. As a systems change leader, you must foster a climate of openness, reflection, and safety.

What Factors Will Influence the Implementation of Systems Change?

By design, systems change embraces complexity and encompasses many levels, innovations, and actors within a system. This complexity only increases the need for careful analysis of the context so that appropriate strategies can be identified, tested, and, if successful, scaled to facilitate progress. You can use implementation science to understand and address the diverse factors that will influence your systems change efforts.

A wide variety of factors (aka facilitators and barriers, determinants) have been shown to influence innovation implementation. Several frameworks define the range of relevant factors. The widely used Consolidated Framework for Implementation Research[25,26] (CFIR; Table 10.1) defines five domains and specific constructs shown to influence implementation, including: (a) the characteristics of the individuals involved in implementation (including those receiving the innovation); (b) the characteristics of the innovations; (c) the inner context; (d) the outer context; and (e) the implementation

TABLE 10.1 Key Factors Influencing Change Implementation

DOMAIN	DEFINITION
Intervention characteristics	Characteristics of the intervention being implemented in a specific setting, including the interventions core components and the adaptable elements, structures, and systems related to the intervention and the setting where it is being implemented
Characteristics of individuals	Individuals who are involved with the intervention and/or implementation process who have opinions, beliefs, and agency to take action, all of which influence implementation
Outer setting	The economic, political, and social context within which an organization resides
Inner setting	Features of structural, political, and cultural contexts through which the implementation process will proceed
Implementation process	An interrelated series of sub processes that do not necessarily occur sequentially and may be progressing simultaneously at multiple levels of an organization

Sources: Data from Damschroder LJ, Aron DC, Keith RE, et al. Fostering implementation of health services research findings into practice: a consolidated framework for advancing implementation science. *Implement Sci.* 2009;4:50. doi:10.1186/1748-5908-4-50; Michie S, Johnston M, Abraham C, et al. Making psychological theory useful for implementing evidence-based practice: a consensus approach. *Qual Saf Health Care.* 2005;14(1):26–33. doi:10.1136/qshc.2004.011155.

process. The breadth and depth of the framework make it a valuable resource for understanding the context of the change.

You can apply the CFIR to explore potential influences on any prioritized innovation. For example, you can use it to make sense of focus group data describing partners' past collaborative experiences. The breadth of the framework can help you to capture the diversity of factors at play in your context (e.g., poor communication, limited leadership) while the five domains facilitate concise summarization and communication of major themes. You can work with collaborators to use the findings to develop and refine implementation plans and strategies.

The Theoretical Domains Framework (TDF; Table 10.2)[27,28] unifies diverse behavioral theories related to individual behavioral change. The framework provides a useful guide for understanding and developing strategies to influence individual behavior within a complex system.[29] Individual change—on the part of a service recipient, a service provider, an administrator, a policy maker, a process facilitator, and so forth is at the center of most systems change. You can use the TDF to carefully consider the specific levers to motivate change and guide your choice of strategies to address the factors inhibiting change.[30] For example, cash incentives may encourage and facilitate certain behaviors but may be less acceptable to some actors and challenging to sustain without political commitment and secure financing.[31]

TABLE 10.2 Theoretical Domains Framework

Knowledge (an awareness of the existence of something)

Skills (an ability or proficiency acquired through practice)

Social/professional role and identity (a coherent set of behaviors and displayed personal qualities of an individual in a social or work setting)

Beliefs about capabilities (acceptance of the truth, reality, or validity about an ability, talent, or facility that a person can put to constructive use)

Optimism (the confidence that things will happen for the best or that desired goals will be attained)

Beliefs about consequences (acceptance of the truth, reality, or validity about outcomes of a behavior in a given situation)

Reinforcement (increasing the probability of a response by arranging a dependent relationship, or contingency, between the response and a given stimulus)

Intentions (a conscious decision to perform a behavior or a resolve to act in a certain way)

Goals (mental representations of outcomes or end states that an individual wants to achieve)

Memory, attention, and decision processes (the ability to retain information, focus selectively on aspects of the environment, and choose between two or more alternatives)

Environmental context and resources (any circumstance of a person's situation or environment that discourages or encourages the development of skills and abilities, independence, social competence, and adaptive behavior)

Social influences (those interpersonal processes that can cause individuals to change their thoughts, feelings, or behaviors)

Sources: Data from Michie S, Johnston M, Abraham C, et al. Making psychological theory useful for implementing evidence-based practice: a consensus approach. *Qual Saf Health Care*. 2005;14(1):26–33. doi:10.1136/qshc.2004.011155; Atkins L, Francis J, Islam R, et al. A guide to using the Theoretical Domains Framework of behaviour change to investigate implementation problems. *Implement Sci*. 2017;12(1):77. doi:10.1186/s13012-017-0605-9.

The CFIR and the TDF are just two relevant frameworks that you may find useful for understanding the context of the change. With your change leadership team, you should reflect carefully on the relevance and potential value of using a specific framework and consider the availability of supportive resources (e.g., technical guides, tools, technical assistance). Additional resources for identifying and selecting contextually relevant frameworks are listed in the following.

Why Is Understanding the Context So Important?

Regardless of the framework you use, it is critical that you understand the context in which you are working. As described earlier, you can begin this work in the exploration stage and continue into later stages. This has many important benefits. First, by working with diverse stakeholders to assess the context, you can identify complementary as well as competing perspectives. Left unexplored, competing perspectives might cause conflict among change leaders or cause you to miss opportunities for synergistic efforts. Exploring these factors together can help you and your counterparts generate valuable insights that can help to refine your goals, focus, and scope.

Second, efforts to understand the context provide change leaders like you with opportunities to listen and learn. You can demonstrate a respect for and sincere curiosity about the lives and experiences of actors within the system. In addition to the insights you gather, the relationships that you form and strengthen through this work are a resource that can sustain and support the change effort over time. In systems with a history of discrimination and marginalization, your sincere efforts to understand diverse perspectives and experiences can contribute to the co-creation of a more equitable, just, and effective system.

Finally, taking the time to understand the context informs the selection of specific strategies that you will use to advance the work.[32] Without understanding the system's history, culture, relationships, and resources, you may invest significant time and resources in approaches that are unnecessary, redundant, or even harmful. For example, a past failure with an innovation might be seen by some as evidence of a lack of staff commitment or capacity. Left unexplored, you might choose to avoid similar efforts. However, through a more thorough discussion with a broader range of stakeholders, you might uncover that the failure resulted from a lack of investment in organizational policy and supportive management. You could then work with your counterparts to focus on strengthening support and avoiding such mistakes for future changes.

CREATING AN ENABLING CONTEXT FOR SYSTEMS CHANGE

The third element of the active implementation formula is the Enabling Context. This is perhaps the most compelling yet challenging element, one with special significance for systems change work. Creating an enabling environment requires you to embrace adaptive challenges where both the cause and the solution are unclear. As described by Senge et al.,[1] this depends on your creative, humble, and sustained leadership to foster trust, courage, and compassion among collaborators to tackle challenging issues, such as a community's history of racism and marginalization of specific groups. As a leader, you will need to build collaborative processes that engage diverse stakeholders and foster learning about community, as explored in the following.

How Can I Engage Diverse Stakeholders in Systems Change?

Involving diverse stakeholders in the design, contextualization, and operationalization of systems change has many benefits. First, it is warranted on ethical grounds. The Principles of the Ethical Practice of Public Health[33] emphasizes the importance of community input in policy and program design, delivery, and evaluation. You may have heard the saying "Nothing for us, without us," which captures the spirit of this ethical principle. Second, broad participation enhances the likelihood that the root causes of the challenges experienced by the community will be identified. Sustained dialogue among stakeholders can help you to create new, shared perspectives that can be used to create new solutions. Finally, ongoing collaboration among diverse stakeholders can help you tailor innovations to the context, increasing their fit and feasibility over time. You can ensure that an innovation's "customers" are actively involved across the stages and that your collective decisions respond to the context and the specific needs of the population.[34]

Robust and sustained stakeholder engagement can itself be a systems change innovation, requiring your commitment and sustained effort. You can use your knowledge of the culture and history of the system to initiate action. For example, you could leverage an existing collaborative partnership as a starting point while laying the groundwork for expanded participation among groups that have historically been left out. The International Association of Public Participation has defined a spectrum of public participation that you can use to define and carry out a variety of engagement strategies over the lifetime of your effort (Figure 10.4).[35] Additional practical resources to support stakeholder definition and prioritization are included in the Supplemental Resources list.

	INFORM	CONSULT	INVOLVE	COLLABORATE	EMPOWER
PUBLIC PARTICIPATION GOAL	To provide the public with balanced and objective information to assist them in understanding the problem, alternatives, opportunities and/or solutions.	To obtain public feedback on analysis, alternatives and/or decisions.	To work directly with the public throughout the process to ensure that public concerns and aspirations are consistently understood and considered.	To partner with the public in each aspect of the decision including the development of alternatives and the identification of the preferred solution.	To place final decision making in the hands of the public.
PROMISE TO THE PUBLIC	We will keep you informed.	We will keep you informed, listen to and acknowledge concerns and aspirations, and provide feedback on how public input influenced the decision.	We will work with you to ensure that your concerns and aspirations are directly reflected in the alternatives developed and provide feedback on how public input influenced the decision.	We will look to you for advice and innovation in formulating solutions and incorporate your advice and recommendations into the decisions to the maximum extent possible.	We will implement what you decide.

INCREASING IMPACT ON THE DECISION →

Figure 10.4 Spectrum of public participation.
Source: Reproduced with permission from International Association for Public Participation. Core Values, Ethics, Spectrum—The 3 Pillars of Public Participation. International Association for Public Participation website. https://www.iap2.org/page/pillars. Accessed January 18, 2021.

How Can I Support Continuous Learning?

We build collaborative groups to foster continuous learning for systems change in the face of ongoing and unpredictable change. The authors of the Dynamic Sustainability Framework[36] argue that every aspect of a system is in flux simultaneously, and therefore leaders must adopt a dynamic learning approach. Such an approach means that rather than seeking to exert control over the change, you embrace it. Rather than settle for innovations that are a poor fit for the context, you adopt continuous quality improvement strategies to steadily improve innovation fit and sustainability in the host system. The broad engagement described earlier supports this approach by facilitating collaborative data collection and analysis as well as collective problem-solving. Establishing a shared commitment to learning supported with concrete practices contributes to greater impact and sustainability.

The complex nature of systems change work presents you with multiple learning opportunities. The specific questions that you will face include: Who needs to be involved to help us understand the need? How can we strengthen our capacity to effectively respond? Where can we improve our performance? And how can we expand reach and sustain impact? What's more, technical and adaptive challenges will emerge as you progress, requiring you to reconsider previous assumptions and decisions. The dynamism inherent in these efforts justifies a continuous learning approach.

In summary, implementation science provides conceptual and practical tools that can help you develop and apply the core capabilities of the systems leaders to realize systems change for improved public health. First, you can use implementation frameworks, such as the active implementation stages, to make visible the often implicit and poorly understood decision-making processes of our public health system. These resources can also help you to build shared language and methods among diverse stakeholders. Second, you can apply available resources, including the CFIR and TDF, to identify and respond to the most critical factors influencing system performance in the context. Finally, a deeper understanding of the system and the key facilitators and barriers at play can inform an expanded understanding of the stakeholders who should be at the table. Systems leaders can use these lessons from implementation science to foster and sustain the co-creative problem-solving needed to solve complex systems challenges.

CHAPTER SUMMARY

If systems leadership is still dawning, its integration with implementation science is also in its infancy. Systems leaders can use the lessons of implementation science to plan, support, and improve complex systems change efforts. Implementation science is the study *and* application of methods to promote the systematic uptake of and effective use of evidence-based interventions and other innovations to improve population health and well-being.[2-4] This chapter highlights the potential application of key concepts to advance practice in three domains: *Effective Innovations*, *Effective Implementation*, and *Enabling Context*. Implementation science incorporates a systems perspective, increasing the utility of the research for systems change efforts.

Key Messages

- Deciding what to do to address identified needs is a key part of systems change. Multiple innovations may be needed, including structured approaches to organizing, managing, and improving collaborative change efforts.
- Evidence-based frameworks and tools can be used to organize, plan, and support multiple innovations involved in a complex systems change effort.
- Change efforts depend on a supportive environment defined by trust, collaboration, and ongoing learning.

Tips

- Take time to carefully appraise the innovations intended to foster productive change in your system.
- Use implementation competency frameworks to assess and improve workforce capacity in support of prioritized changes.
- Use evidence-based implementation resources and tools (see Supplemental Resources) to support public health systems change efforts.
- Integrate robust stakeholder collaboration and continuous learning through all stages of implementation.

Supplemental Resources

- The Active Implementation Hub: https://nirn.fpg.unc.edu/ai-hub
- The Hexagon Tool: https://nirn.fpg.unc.edu/resources/hexagon-exploration-tool
- Centers for Disease Control and Prevention Policy Analysis Guide: www.cdc.gov/policy/polaris/policyprocess/policy_analysis.html
- Center for Effective Services Guide to Implementation: http://implementation.effectiveservices.org
- Strategic Doing: https://strategicdoing.net
- Consolidated Framework for Implementation Research guide: https://cfirguide.org
- Dissemination and Implementation Models in Health Research and Practice: https://dissemination-implementation.org

REFERENCES

1. Senge P, Hamilton H, Kania J. The dawn of system leadership. *Stanf Soc Innov Rev.* 2015;13(1):27–33. doi:10.48558/YTE7-XT62.
2. Fixsen D, Naoom SF, Blase KA, Friedman RM, Wallace F. *Implementation Research: A Synthesis of the Literature.* 1st ed. University of South Florida, Louis de la Parte Florida Mental Health Institute; 2005:1–125.

3. Rabin BA, Brownson RC, Haire-Joshu D, Kreuter MW, Weaver NL. A glossary for dissemination and implementation research in health. *J Public Health Manag Pract.* 2008;14(2):117–123. doi:10.1097/01.PHH.0000311888.06252.bb.

4. Eccles MP, Mittman BS. Welcome to implementation science. *Implement Sci.* 2006;1(1):1. doi:10.1186/1748-5908-1-1.

5. Institute of Medicine (US) Committee. *Crossing the quality chasm: a new health system for the 21st century.* National Academies Press (US) 2001:1–364. doi:10.17226/10027.

6. Nilsen P. Making sense of implementation theories, models and frameworks. *Implement Sci.* 2015;10:53. doi:10.1186/s13012-015-0242-0.

7. Easterling D, Metz A. Getting real with strategy: insights from implementation science. *Foundation Rev.* 2016;8(2).

8. Evidence Tools. MCH Evidence Center website. https://www.mchevidence.org/tools/. Accessed March 25, 2021.

9. The California Evidence-Based Clearinghouse for Child Welfare. https://www.cebc4cw .org/. Accessed March 25, 2021.

10. AMCHP Innovation Station. Association of Maternal & Child Health Programs website. http://www.amchp.org/programsandtopics/BestPractices/InnovationStation/Pages/ Innovation-Station.aspx. Accessed December 27, 2020.

11. What Works for Health. County Health Rankings & Roadmaps website. https://www .countyhealthrankings.org/take-action-to-improve-health/what-works-for-health. Accessed March 25, 2021.

12. Kania J, Kramer M. Collective impact. *SSIR.* 2011 Winter;9(1):36–41. doi:10.48558/ 5900-KN19.

13. Spoth R, Greenberg M, Bierman K, Redmond C. PROSPER community-university partnership model for public education systems: capacity-building for evidence-based, competence-building prevention. *Prev Sci.* 2004;5(1):31–39. doi:10.1023/B:PREV.000 0013979.52796.8b.

14. Friedman M. *Trying Hard Is Not Good Enough. 10th Anniversary.* PARSE Publishing; 2015.

15. Strategic Doing: Do More Together. https://strategicdoing.net/. Accessed January 18, 2021.

16. Metz A, Bartley L. Active implementation frameworks for program success. *Zero Three.* 2012;32(4):11–18.

17. Aarons GA, Hurlburt M, Horwitz SM. Advancing a conceptual model of evidence-based practice implementation in public service sectors. *Adm Policy Ment Health.* 2011;38(1): 4–23. doi:10.1007/s10488-010-0327-7.

18. Meyers DC, Durlak JA, Wandersman A. The quality implementation framework: a synthesis of critical steps in the implementation process. *Am J Community Psychol.* 2012;50(3– 4):462–480. doi:10.1007/s10464-012-9522-x.

19. Metz A, Burke K, Albers B, Louison L, Bartley L. *A Practice Guide to Supporting Implementation.* University of North Carolina at Chapel Hill, Chapel Hill, North Carolina. 2020.

20. Saldana L, Chamberlain P. Supporting implementation: the role of community development teams to build infrastructure. *Am J Community Psychol.* 2012;50(3–4):334–346. doi:10.1007/ s10464-012-9503-0.

21. Chamberlain P, Roberts R, Jones H, Marsenich L, Sosna T, Price JM. Three collaborative models for scaling up evidence-based practices. *Adm Policy Ment Health.* 2012;39(4):278– 290. doi:10.1007/s10488-011-0349-9.

22. Hurlburt M, Aarons GA, Fettes D, Willging C, Gunderson L, Chaffin MJ. Interagency collaborative team model for capacity building to scale-up evidence-based practice. *Child Youth Serv Rev.* 2014;39:160–168. doi:10.1016/j.childyouth.2013.10.005.

23. Joyce B, Showers B. *Student Achievement Through Staff Development.* Designing Training and Peer Coaching: Our Needs for Learning; 2002:1–5.

24. Wells R, Yates L, Morgan I, deRosset L, Cilenti D. Using the Wilder Collaboration Factors Inventory to strengthen collaborations for improving maternal and child health. *Matern Child Health J.* 2021 Mar;25(3):377–384. doi:10.1007/s10995-020-03091-2.

25. Damschroder LJ, Aron DC, Keith RE, Kirsh SR, Alexander JA, Lowery JC. Fostering implementation of health services research findings into practice: a consolidated framework for advancing implementation science. *Implement Sci.* 2009;4:50. doi:10.1186/1748-5908-4-50.

26. Kirk MA, Kelley C, Yankey N, Birken SA, Abadie B, Damschroder L. A systematic review of the use of the Consolidated Framework for Implementation Research. *Implement Sci.* 2016;11:72. doi:10.1186/s13012-016-0437-z.

27. Michie S, Johnston M, Abraham C, et al. Making psychological theory useful for implementing evidence based practice: a consensus approach. *Qual Saf Health Care.* 2005;14(1):26–33. doi:10.1136/qshc.2004.011155.

28. Cane J, O'Connor D, Michie S. Validation of the theoretical domains framework for use in behaviour change and implementation research. *Implement Sci.* 2012;7:37. doi:10.1186/1748-5908-7-37.

29. Atkins L, Francis J, Islam R, et al. A guide to using the Theoretical Domains Framework of behaviour change to investigate implementation problems. *Implement Sci.* 2017;12(1):77. doi:10.1186/s13012-017-0605-9.

30. French SD, Green SE, O'Connor DA, et al. Developing theory-informed behaviour change interventions to implement evidence into practice: A systematic approach using the Theoretical Domains Framework. *Implement Sci.* 2012 Apr 24;7:38. doi:10.1186/1748-5908-7-38.

31. Beidas RS, Becker-Haimes EM, Adams DR, et al. Feasibility and acceptability of two incentive-based implementation strategies for mental health therapists implementing cognitive-behavioral therapy: a pilot study to inform a randomized controlled trial. *Implement Sci.* 2017;12(1):148. doi:10.1186/s13012-017-0684-7.

32. Nilsen P, Bernhardsson S. Context matters in implementation science: a scoping review of determinant frameworks that describe contextual determinants for implementation outcomes. *BMC Health Serv Res.* 2019;19(1):189. doi:10.1186/s12913-019-4015-3.

33. Thomas JC, Sage MS, Dillenberg JD, Guillory JG. A code of ethics for public health. *Am J Public Health.* 2002;92(7):1057–1059.

34. Cabassa LJ. Implementation science: why it matters for the future of social work. *J Soc Work Educ.* 2016;52(Suppl 1):S38–S50. doi:10.1080/10437797.2016.1174648.

35. Core Values, Ethics, Spectrum—The 3 Pillars of Public Participation. International Association for Public Participation website. https://www.iap2.org/page/pillars. Accessed January 18, 2021.

36. Chambers DA, Glasgow RE, Stange KC. The dynamic sustainability framework: addressing the paradox of sustainment amid ongoing change. *Implement Sci.* 2013;8:117. doi:10.1186/1748-5908-8-117.

11

Sustainability and Effective Public Health: A Committed Relationship

Gillian Gawne-Mittelstaedt

CHAPTER OBJECTIVES

At the end of this chapter, the practitioner will be able to:

※ Recognize the range of ideas and concepts found within public health's definitions of sustainability.
※ Identify and distinguish among actions, behaviors, and traits associated with sustainable public health programs.
※ Recognize several common facilitators and barriers to sustainability.
※ Be able to apply a sustainability lens to their current programs and initiatives.

INTRODUCTION

Sustainability is a fundamental building block of systems change and a cornerstone of effective public health. Sustainability is, in fact, so intertwined with effective public health that it could be said that they are (*or should be*) in a committed relationship. As a public health practitioner, you have inevitably encountered barriers to sustainability in your work and may have even seen an untimely ending of a good initiative (or two or three). When this happens, and you experience a loss of critical programs or services in which you are personally invested, it can be disheartening. The dissolution of a program can be an opportunity for learning, however, through reflection and evaluation. It is also an opportunity for systems leadership, as you engage your colleagues in exploring how to build sustainability more explicitly in future initiatives.

This chapter introduces the core concepts of sustainability in public health, with the proposition that sustainability is not an endpoint but a way of operating. Shediac-Rizkallah and Bone[1] suggest that sustainability needs to be a planned approach rather than a latent goal. Successful programs, they observe, operate with sustainability as a dynamic process, versus a static endpoint. This chapter explores these ideas, introducing practical sustainability concepts for your systems leadership toolbox.

FRAMING SUSTAINABILITY: WHY IT MATTERS FOR PUBLIC HEALTH SUCCESS

Effective public health programs are a success not because they sustain, but because by sustaining, they improve the lives of not just a few individuals but of entire communities. Achieving population-scale impacts is just one reason why sustainability is integral to systems-level reform. Other reasons why public health programs need to be sustained over time include:

1. **Implementing policy, systems, and environmental (PSE) change often requires years**, or decades, to take full effect. Time is particularly important as PSE changes are complex, adaptive challenges and address multiple causal factors that require prolonged effort.[2]
2. **Long-term impacts may not be evident for several years**, especially where behavior change is involved and there is a latency period required.[3] Many health promotion programs, such as tobacco cessation, require sustained implementation. As an example, the Community Intervention Trial for Smoking Cessation (COMMIT) did not begin to see results in smoking cessation until 3 years after the communities were randomized.[4] Roussos and Fawcett[5] observe that change in population health outcomes, "in most community health areas may not be detectable for 3 to 10 years after the beginning of programs."[5(p374)]
3. **Programs and interventions require significant public investment**, both monetary and nonmonetary. Discontinued programs and partnerships, particularly those with promising results, are not supportive of good fiscal stewardship if they are not sustained after the initial investment.[3]

DEFINITIONS: THE MANY DIMENSIONS OF SUSTAINABILITY

In a literal interpretation, sustainability is a measure of duration, but when applied to public health, sustainability is multidimensional. It is akin to a tree, with a branch for sustainability of institutions and organizations, a branch for sustainability of programs and interventions, and a branch for sustainability of partnerships and collaborations. As with any organic entity, sustainability is not permanent, but is an iterative, constant process of adaptation and change. At its core, sustainability is less an outcome and more a way of achieving an outcome.

Many definitions of sustainability reflect the idea that sustainability is more than duration. Yet there is little agreement as to what sustainability does encompass. In academic literature, there is no unified conceptual understanding of sustainability. Shelton et al.,[6] in a review of the public health literature on sustainability, concluded: "Despite a growing interest in research on sustainability, the literature has been highly fragmented across topical areas and disciplines. Most notably, until recently, the field has lacked a common set of definitions, research questions, measures, and conceptual frameworks."[6(p57)] In a systematic review of the sustainability literature among community health collaboratives, Hearld et al.[7] reviewed 42 eligible studies and found that over 40% did not explicitly define sustainability. Of those that did define sustainability, just over a third utilized only a basic and broad definition of sustainability.

Despite the variability, there are several recurring ideas that appear in definitions of sustainability, including adaptability, collaboration, resilience, and resources. Figure 11.1 summarizes these four elements and how they relate to definitions of sustainability.

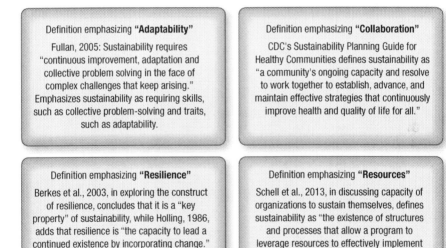

Definition emphasizing **"Adaptability"**

Fullan, 2005: Sustainability requires "continuous improvement, adaptation and collective problem solving in the face of complex challenges that keep arising." Emphasizes sustainability as requiring skills, such as collective problem-solving and traits, such as adaptability.

Definition emphasizing **"Collaboration"**

CDC's Sustainability Planning Guide for Healthy Communities defines sustainability as "a community's ongoing capacity and resolve to work together to establish, advance, and maintain effective strategies that continuously improve health and quality of life for all."

Definition emphasizing **"Resilience"**

Berkes et al., 2003, in exploring the construct of resilience, concludes that it is a "key property" of sustainability, while Holling, 1986, adds that resilience is "the capacity to lead a continued existence by incorporating change."

Definition emphasizing **"Resources"**

Schell et al., 2013, in discussing capacity of organizations to sustain themselves, defines sustainability as "the existence of structures and processes that allow a program to leverage resources to effectively implement and maintain evidence-based policies and activities."

Figure 11.1 Varied elements in the definitions of sustainability.

Sources: Fullan M. *Leadership and Sustainability.* Corwin; 2005; Batan M, Butterfoss FD, Jaffe A, LaPier T. *Healthy Communities Program: Sustainability Planning Guide.* Centers for Disease Control and Prevention; n.d.; Berkes F, Colding J, Folke C, eds. *Navigating Social–Ecological Systems: Building Resilience for Complexity and Change.* Cambridge University Press; 2003; Holling CS. The resilience of terrestrial ecosystems: local surprise and global change. In: Clark WC, Munn RE, eds. *Sustainable Development of the Biosphere.* Cambridge University Press; 1986:292–317; Schell SF, Luke DA, Schooley MW, et al. Public health program capacity for sustainability: a new framework. *Implement Sci.* 2013;8:15. doi:10.1186/1748-5908-8-15.

The authors of these sustainability definitions have each sought to describe what sustainability looks like once it exists. Yet an even more pressing and perpetual question for researchers and practitioners alike is "How do we *get* to sustainability in the first place?" Answering this question requires "getting off the dance floor and going to the balcony."[8] The balcony perspective, a systems leadership tool, is particularly useful for exploring the topic of sustainability in our work.

Exercise

Stepping back (or *up*) to the balcony, take a few minutes to experiment with this perspective by applying it to one of your programs or initiatives: What factors appear to facilitate or inhibit the sustainability of your current programs? List as many factors as you can identify, then take a second pass at your notes, using the four definitions of sustainability in Figure 11.1 as an analytic lens. Apply the following questions to your observations:

1. Is there evidence of *adaptability* in the program, such as collective program-solving? In what ways has your program adapted to meet changing circumstances?
2. What actions or behaviors did you see in your organization that built *resilience*?
3. Are *resources* other than the initial funding source leveraged to ensure program stability and survival?
4. What role did *collaboration* with partners have in facilitating or inhibiting your program sustainability?

GETTING TO SUSTAINABILITY: LESSONS FROM PUBLIC HEALTH PRACTITIONERS

Very few innovations start out institutionalized, or with permanent funding, so there is great interest in understanding precisely how programs get to sustainability. Close observers recognize that sustainability is a product of what people and organizations do, but it is also a product of *how* people and organizations do what they do. To illustrate, an organization that develops a strategic plan, conducts a program evaluation, or pursues Medicaid reimbursement for their program is taking an action, with the intent of producing new knowledge or resources to sustain their program. In contrast, an organization that exhibits certain behaviors, such as transparent communication about resources, or purposeful strategic management, is creating a dynamic culture that fuels sustainability. Evidence suggests that both actions and behaviors are necessary and that when combined, they act as drivers of sustainability. Researchers who study these actions and behaviors have developed sustainability frameworks to help explain the drivers and their relationship to one another. In Figure 11.2, four sustainability frameworks are shown, from four different sources and perspectives. A degree of commonality is seen across the frameworks, illustrating how certain actions and behaviors are consistently associated with sustainability.

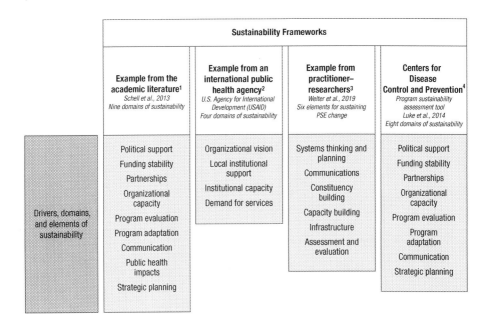

Figure 11.2 Sustainability frameworks.

[1]The research conducted by Schell et al.[9] that resulted in this framework included a comprehensive review of the literature and concept mapping.

[2]The USAID elements were identified as "prerequisites for sustainability" among institutions, adding that sustainability also required becoming independent of grants.

[3]The University of Illinois Chicago School of Public Health, in collaboration with the Cook County Department of Public Health, identified these drivers while helping organizations and communities plan for implementation and sustainability of policy, systems, and environmental change.

[4]The Centers for Disease Control and Prevention funded research[10] to test the validity of the Program Sustainability Assessment Tool (PSAT), which identifies key domains of sustainability.

Sources: Schell SF, Luke DA, Schooley MW, et al. Public health program capacity for sustainability: a new framework. *Implement Sci.* 2013;8:15. doi:10.1186/1748-5908-8-15; Committee on Public Health Strategies to Improve Health & Institute of Medicine. *For the Public's Health: Investing in a Healthier Future.* National Academies Press (US); 2012. http://www.ncbi.nlm.nih.gov/books/NBK201023/; Welter C, Jarpe-Ratner E, Massuda Barnett G, et al. Key drivers of success: what catalyzes lasting change in your organization or community? *Action Learning Brief No. 003.* Illinois Prevention Research Center, University of Illinois Chicago; April 2019. https://illinoisprc.org/publications/; Luke DA, Calhoun A, Robichaux CB, Elliott MB, Moreland-Russell S. The program sustainability assessment tool: a new instrument for public health programs. *Prev Chronic Dis.* 2014;11:130184. doi:10.5888/pcd11.130184.

In Figure 11.2, actions and behaviors are highlighted as separate concepts, yet in practice they exist in a close relationship. An action conducted repeatedly, such as evaluating a program, eventually becomes a behavior, such as strategic management. Rather than categories such as actions and behaviors, it may be more apt to conceive of sustainability as a systems leadership mindset, a way of thinking that permeates one's work. Donald Schon[11] describes this mindset and how it is fundamental to sustainability:

> *"We must . . . become adept at learning. We must become able not only to transform our institutions, in response to changing situations and requirements; we must invest and develop institutions which are 'learning systems,' that is to say, systems capable of bringing about their own continuing transformation."*[11(p74)]

Exercise

Review the four sustainability frameworks in Figure 11.2. On a separate piece of paper, create a column for a fifth framework. Choose a public health program, initiative, or coalition with which you are most familiar in terms of its history. Reflecting on that program, create your own framework, listing as many sustainability actions or behaviors as you have observed. For the actions that you identify, explore *how* and *why* those sustainability actions were conducted. For example, if you wrote, "We built political support with local leaders," reflect on *how* you built the political support. Where you noted sustainability actions, reflect on the precursors that led your organization or coalition to take these sustainability actions in the first place. This will provide clues about the organizational culture and behaviors that you will have to address when championing sustainability.

SUSTAINABILITY FACILITATORS AND BARRIERS

While there are myriad factors that impact sustainability, there are several facilitators and barriers that appear frequently in both academic and grey literature (Figure 11.3).

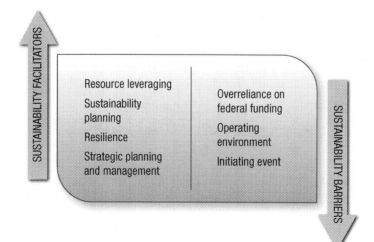

Figure 11.3 Sustainability facilitators and barriers.

Sustainability Facilitators

1. ***Resource Leveraging.*** The ability to leverage resources, both monetary and nonmonetary, is a well-recognized facilitator of sustainability. Towe et al.,[12] in observing sustainability among community health collaborations, found that the need for financial maintenance was coupled with the need for nonfiscal investment (e.g., leadership commitment and stakeholder buy-in). Programs and initiatives that endure over time are shown to have strategically designed their funding and resource efforts. Consider the strategic plans that your organization or coalition produces: Do the plans focus on outcome measures only, such as a reduction in disease prevalence, or do they also include process measures, such as building adequate resources for long-term program operation? If process measures are not included in your organization's strategic plan, what opportunities exist to raise this gap among your colleagues?

2. ***Sustainability Planning.*** Pilot programs and new interventions require an evidence base, which drives an initial focus on data collection and measurement of outcomes. The conversation about sustaining a program, once it has shown itself to be effective, often does not begin for several years. By this time, the initial grant period may be over, and the influx of resources may have waned. When sustainability is not conceived of until after the planning, implementation, and evaluation phases, a program can be precarious. In *Factors That Predict Financial Sustainability of Community Coalitions*,[13] researchers observed 14 partnerships over a 5-year period, interviewing 164 team members and 10 prevention coordinators. While all 14 community teams were still in existence after 5 years, they found "substantial variability in the amount of funds raised, and these differences were predicted by earlier and concurrent team functioning and by team *sustainability planning*."[13(p158)] In the End Games report,[14] private foundations were interviewed about the sustainability of the initiatives they funded. Many recommended that a focus on sustainability "should come earlier" and that sustainability "should be part of the original design" of an initiative.[14(p18)] The concept of planning for sustainability is intuitive, yet not widely practiced. What opportunities exist for you to introduce sustainability planning into your organization or coalition?

3. ***Resilience.*** Resilience is shown to be a key facilitator of sustainability and is best described as "the incremental capacity of an organization to anticipate and adjust to the environment."[15(p1617)] Resilience is also understood as the capability to revive one's organization over time, through innovation and re-invention. Building resilience into public health programs is an ongoing developmental task, yet one that does not occur spontaneously. It requires building several competencies, including the capacity to (a) anticipate potential change and disruption to a program, (b) cope with change and disruption as it occurs, and then (c) adapt accordingly. To anticipate, cope with, and adapt to change are thus tantamount to sustainability and are closely related to systems leadership. In the "Dawn of Systems Leadership," Senge et al.[16] describe how systems leaders shift the "collective focus from reactive problem solving to co-creating the future."[16(p15)] Reflecting on the culture and behaviors in your own organization, what actions have you

observed that indicate adaptability and resilience? How does your organization anticipate, cope with, or adapt to funding disruption?

4. ***Strategic Planning and Strategic Management.*** Ways that organizations effectively anticipate, cope with, and adapt to change are through strategic planning and strategic management. While creating a planning document can feel like a rote exercise, public health leaders recognize that strategic planning creates a space for thinking about systems complexity and preparing for disruption within that system. As Bryson[17] notes, strategic planning is a method for cultivating "strategic thought and action," which enhances an organization's capacity to respond to change. And an organization's capacity to respond to change is a key pathway to sustainability. Strategic management, the process of continual analysis, monitoring, planning, and evaluation, is equally important to sustainability. With an emphasis on real-time feedback and cycles of organizational learning, strategic management helps organizations anticipate, cope with, and adapt to change.

Sustainability Barriers

1. ***Overreliance on Federal Resources.*** In public health, it is difficult to conduct a program or initiative without at least some degree of federal funding. Yet federal funds, when relied upon too heavily, can become a barrier to long-term program sustainability. With the ebb and flow of federal resources, being reliant upon federal funds can be "a risky strategy."[18] In addition to year-over-year fluctuations in funding levels, grant programs can be unpredictable. Discretionary public health funding can pivot quickly when a new public health crisis or emergency takes place. This instability stunts the permanence of public health programs, particularly when those programs are not yet institutionalized or embedded. Researchers have observed that the end of a federal grant not only contributes to the end of a program but may even contribute to the end of sustainability efforts in general. Pluye et al.[3] reflected on this phenomenon, observing: "In our opinion, when the continuation of programs is far beyond the means of the community, the end of external financing does not represent the beginning of a sustainability phase but leads to the end of the sustainability process."[3(126)] Though *many* initiatives rely on a singular funding source, dialogue around this reality in your workplace can be a precursor to building a more diverse, stable funding base.

2. ***Operating Environment.*** Funding may be a barrier to sustainability, yet there are other factors within the larger operating environment that affect the sustainability of public health programs. Changes in public health take place in a context that involves political support or, at a minimum, political tolerance. Yet public acceptance for innovative programs often lags and can be a barrier to widespread adoption, such as taxation on soft drinks or tobacco-free multifamily housing. In addition to political shifts, social, economic, and environmental forces impact the public health operating environment. Coronavirus disease 2019 (COVID-19), climate change, and surging homelessness are 21st-century examples that have strained the U.S. economy, and in turn, created competition for congressional

attention. However, the level of funding is only part of the barrier to sustainability. The 2012 report "For the Public's Health: Investing in a Healthier Future" by the Institute of Medicine investigated funding within the public health system and identified insufficient funding but also remarked upon the "dysfunction in how the public health infrastructure is funded, organized, and equipped to use its funding."[19(p2)] The report also identified that the operating environment in which public health programs are funded can be a barrier to sustainability, describing it as a "patchwork of funding streams, purposes, and funding mechanisms."[19(p51)]

3. ***Initiating Event.*** Public health programs are frequently initiated as pilots, with a grant to test their feasibility and efficacy. Similarly, coalitions are often initiated by a granting agency that requires the formation of a coalition or partnership. In both situations, regardless of how successful the program or coalition becomes, when the initiating event is a grant, sustainability can be a challenge. Mays and Schutchfield,[20] in exploring the performance of multisector public health partnerships, observed the unintended consequences of pilot-focused funding: "Funds are usually allocated for a limited time and come with many regulations. There is often not enough money to go beyond the pilot. Pilot projects too often remain just that."[20(p2)] Researchers of implementation science, a growing field in public health, have evaluated why some programs move from pilot to permanence, while others demonstrate value yet cease to exist after their initiating grant. They found that sustainable programs and partnerships demonstrate three traits in particular: securing broad support, demonstrating their value, and leveraging resources. These traits are evident in the following case.

PUTTING SUSTAINABILITY INTO PRACTICE: A PUBLIC HEALTH LEADERSHIP STORY

With each new public health crisis or epidemic, there is a wave of political attention, ushering in new funding opportunities and legislative action. When the wave recedes, initiatives left standing are often those that have embedded themselves through sustainable funding and partnerships. The U.S. Agency for International Development echoes this in its definition of sustainability: "the capacity to maintain program services at a level that will provide ongoing prevention and treatment for a health problem *after termination of major financial, managerial and technical assistance from an external donor.*"[21]

By the end of the 20th century, asthma had become one of the most prevalent chronic diseases in the United States, making it a leading cause of healthcare utilization[22] and a harbinger of the nation's growing health disparities.[23] Around this time, Tracy Enger was working as a program analyst in the Environmental Protection Agency's Indoor Environments Division (IED). IED had no regulatory levers to address asthma, nor were they a public health agency, yet IED was uniquely poised to address a critical asthma risk factor: environmental triggers. A growing body of evidence had established an association among environmental triggers, asthma severity,

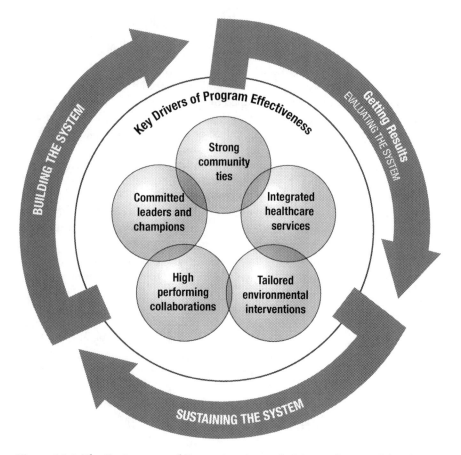

Figure 11.4 The Environmental Protection Agency's drivers of successful asthma programs (the "change package").

and increased healthcare utilization. With the initial waves of federal funding, asthma stakeholders began piloting interventions and building an evidence base. The Asthma Team at IED, demonstrating excellence in leadership, began building a network of asthma champions that could implement systems-level reforms, from clinical medicine and public health to community-based and advocacy organizations. At the same time, they set out to unearth the key drivers behind sustained, successful asthma programs, seeking to understand not only what results were achieved, but how results were achieved. Through research with the University of Michigan Asthma Health Outcomes Project, five key drivers were identified (Figure 11.4), including: (a) strong community ties, (b) integrated healthcare services, (c) tailored environmental interventions, (d) high-performing collaborations, and (e) committed leaders and champions.

To ground their research, Tracy and the Asthma Team compared these five drivers across more than 250 members in their *Communities in Action* network. As supportive evidence grew, they established a goal of recruiting 1,000 new communities to join *Communities in Action* and learn about the Change Package. In doing so, they were building a cadre of organizations trained to think about and prepare for their own sustainability. Tacitly, the Change Package illustrated how sustainability, a process, is foundational to an organization achieving its goals or its outcomes.

Importantly, the Change Package demonstrates that building a program and getting results are phases, not end points. One of the three phases, shown in Figure 11.4, is about "Sustaining the System." By researching asthma programs nationwide, the IED Team was able to discern the specific strategies used by successful asthma programs to sustain their work. These include: Strategy 1—use data to demonstrate your program's value; Strategy 2—be visible, as funders support what they know; Strategy 3—make it easy to support your program; and Strategy 4—promote institutional change for sustainability. Reflecting on one of your recent initiatives, which of these four strategies were you and your partners able to apply? In what ways did your team "make it easy to support your program"? What barriers or facilitators did you encounter to promote sustainability of your program?

In a 2021 interview, Tracy reflected on the strategies that she and her team have observed among sustained, successful asthma programs. They included:

1. Programs and organizations tend to "do what they know." To sustain their programs, asthma champions reflect on their programs to understand how they know what they know. To illustrate, Tracy has seen that those asthma programs sustaining themselves during COVID are those that have reflected on not only what they do, but how they do it, which enables them to pivot when circumstances change. Without this awareness, Tracy adds, programs "might work for a minute, but they're not as likely to work in the long run" (Tracy Enger, personal interview, January 10, 2021).

2. Sustained, successful initiatives are designed with the results in mind. Program champions think about the outcomes they want and what they will need to implement and sustain these outcomes. When programs are not sustained, Tracy suggests it often goes back to building the program with endpoints in mind. "You have programs that start up doing what they know how to do, at a specific moment in time and in response perhaps to an important need, but they develop it without looking at the end picture" (Tracy Enger, personal interview, January 10, 2021).

3. To sustain their program, champions make sure they know exactly *what* they do well, and they continually sell this to partners and funders. They know they have something to offer and ensure their program's value is known.

4. To sustain their program, champions do not take any relationships for granted, but instead work to cultivate and maintain key partnerships.

5. To sustain their program, champions work to recognize when and how their program is evolving; they make evaluation a constant process. Tracy notes, "We see evaluation, but too often—it's too late. We need to build in opportunities to regularly monitor our work and tweak our ingredients if something is missing" (Tracy Enger, personal interview, January 10, 2021).

Exercise

Reflect on a program, initiative, or coalition you were involved with that did not sustain over time. Using an Ishikowa (fishbone) diagram, see how many factors or forces you can identify that appear to have contributed to the lack of sustainability. After you have completed the diagram, reflect on whether these same factors or forces are present in any of your organization's current programs and how you might lead a sustainability conversation to address them.

CHAPTER SUMMARY

In this chapter, we have reviewed core concepts of sustainability in public health, exploring why sustainability is necessary for achieving population-scale outcomes, and for solving complex and adaptive challenges. As illustrated, sustainability is achieved through explicit actions, such as sustainability planning or seeking diverse financial resources before the initiating grant ends. Sustainability is also achieved through institutional capacity and behaviors, such as systems-level thinking, or engaging in strategic management and program evaluation. Knowing how to help your program or organization achieve sustainability is an essential tool of systems leadership. The tools in this chapter, along with the exercises, are designed to help you in this effort.

Key Messages

- Sustainability in public health has no uniform definition, but certain elements appear frequently and are associated with effective, sustained public health programs, including adaptability, collaboration, resources, and resilience.
- There are *actions* that an organization or coalition can take to promote sustainability, including developing a strategic plan, conducting an evaluation, or pursuing non federal resources. There are also *behaviors* that a systems leader can help cultivate within their organization to promote sustainability, including transparent communication, fostering partnerships, and building adaptive capacity.
- While there are many barriers to sustainability, evidence indicates that *planning* for sustainability—explicitly building readiness for change—is an effective strategy for long-term program survival.

Tips

- Prepare for sustainability from the outset, from the program design phase. Do not wait until grant funding is set to expire, but "design with the results in mind."
- As successes become apparent in your program, communicate your program value to key decision-makers and partners. Cultivate a relationship with future partners who might provide monetary or nonmonetary resources to your program once grant funding expires.

- As a systems leader, remember that sustainability is an ongoing dynamic process and that you have tools, such as strategic planning and strategic management, that foster organizational learning and resilience.

Supplemental Resources

- Bringing the Future into Focus: A Step-by-Step Sustainability Planning Workbook. Georgia Health Policy Center: www.ruralhealthinfo.org/sustainability/pdf/bringing-the-future-into-focus-sustainability-planning-workbook.pdf
- Program Sustainability Assessment Tool (PSAT): https://sustaintool.org/
- Sustaining the Work or Initiative: A Toolkit of the Community Toolbox: https://ctb.ku.edu/en/sustaining-work-or-initiative
- A Sustainability Planning Guide for Healthy Communities (Centers for Disease Control and Prevention): www.cdc.gov/nccdphp/dch/programs/healthycommunitiesprogram/pdf/sustainability_guide.pdf
- Key drivers of success: What catalyzes lasting change in your organization or community? Action Learning Brief No. 003. Illinois Prevention Research Center, University of Illinois Chicago: https://p3rc.uic.edu/wp-content/uploads/sites/561/2019/11/ALB3_Key-Drivers_508.pdf

REFERENCES

1. Shediac-Rizkallah MC, Bone LR. Planning for the sustainability of community-based health programs: conceptual frameworks and future directions for research, practice and policy. *Health Educ Res.* 1998;13(1):87–108. doi:10.1093/her/13.1.87.
2. Honeycutt S, Leeman J, McCarthy WJ, et al. Evaluating policy, systems, and environmental change interventions: lessons learned from CDC's prevention research centers. *Prev Chronic Dis.* 2015;12:E174. doi:10.5888/pcd12.150281.
3. Pluye P, Potvin L, Denis J-L. Making public health programs last: conceptualizing sustainability. *Evaluat Prog Plann.* 2004;27(2):121–133. doi:10.1016/j.evalprogplan.2004.01.001.
4. Community Intervention Trial for Smoking Cessation (COMMIT): I. cohort results from a four-year community intervention. *Am J Public Health.*1995 Feb;85(2):183–92. doi:10.2105/ajph.85.2.183.
5. Roussos ST, Fawcett SB. A review of collaborative partnerships as a strategy for improving community health. *Annu Rev Public Health.* 2000;21:369–402. doi:10.1146/annurev.publhealth.21.1.369.
6. Shelton RC, Cooper BR, Stirman SW. The sustainability of evidence-based interventions and practices in public health and health care. *Annu Rev Public Health.* 2018;39(1):55–76. doi:10.1146/annurev-publhealth-040617-014731.
7. Hearld L, Alexander JA, Wolf LJ, Shi Y. Funding profiles of multisector health care alliances and their positioning for sustainability. *J Health Org Manage.* 2018;32(4):587–602. doi:10.1108/JHOM-01-2018-0003.
8. Heifetz RA, Linsky M. A survival guide for leaders. *Harvard Business Review;* June 1, 2002. https://hbr.org/2002/06/a-survival-guide-for-leaders

9. Schell SF, Luke DA, Schooley MW, et al. Public health program capacity for sustainability: a new framework. *Implement Sci.* 2013;8:15. doi:10.1186/1748-5908-8-15.

10. Luke DA, Calhoun A, Robichaux CB, Elliott MB, Moreland-Russell S. The program sustainability assessment tool: a new instrument for public health programs. *Prev Chronic Dis.* 2014;11:130184. doi:10.5888/pcd11.130184.

11. Schon DA. *Beyond the Stable State.* 1st American ed. Random House; 1971.

12. Towe VL, Leviton L, Chandra A, Sloan JC, Tait M, Orleans T. Cross-sector collaborations and partnerships: essential ingredients to help shape health and well-being. *Health Affairs.* 2016;35(11):1964–1969. doi:10.1377/hlthaff.2016.0604.

13. Greenberg MT, Feinberg ME, Johnson LE, Perkins DF, Welsh JA, Spoth RL. Factors that predict financial sustainability of community coalitions: five years of findings from the PROSPER partnership project. *Prev Sci.* 2015;16(1):158–167. doi:10.1007/s11121-014-0483-1.

14. The Annie E. Casey Foundation. End games: The challenge of sustainability. The Annie E. Casey Foundation. https://www.aecf.org/resources/end-games-the-challenge-of-sustainability/. Published April 1, 2002. Accessed January 23, 2021.

15. Ortiz-de-Mandojana N, Bansal P. The long-term benefits of organizational resilience through sustainable business practices. *Strategic Management Journal.* 2015;37(8):1615–1631. doi:10.1002/smj.2410.

16. Senge P, Hamilton H, Kania J. The dawn of system leadership. *Stanf Soc Innov Rev.* 2015;13(1):27–33. doi:10.48558/YTE7-XT62.

17. Bryson JM. A strategic planning process for public and non-profit organizations. *Long Range Plann.* 1988;21(1):73–81. doi:10.1016/0024-6301(88)90061-1.

18. Bingham T, Walters G. Financial sustainability within UK charities: community sport trusts and corporate social responsibility partnerships. *Voluntas.* 2013;24(3):606–629. https://www.jstor.org/stable/42629829.

19. Committee on Public Health Strategies to Improve Health & Institute of Medicine. For the Public's Health: Investing in a Healthier Future. National Academies Press (US); 2012. http://www.ncbi.nlm.nih.gov/books/NBK201023/.

20. Coursey Bailey SB. Focusing on solid partnerships across multiple sectors for population health improvement. *Preventing Chronic Disease.* 2010 November;7(6):A115. PMID: 20950522.

21. U.S. Agency for International Development. Sustainability of development programs: a compendium of donor experience. U.S. Agency for International Development; 1998.

22. Nunes C, Pereira AM, Morais-Almeida M. Asthma costs and social impact. *Asthma Res Pract.* 2017;3:1. doi:10.1186/s40733-016-0029-3.

23. Gold DR, Wright R. Population disparities in asthma. *Annu Rev Public Health.* 2005;26(1):89–113. doi:10.1146/annurev.publhealth.26.021304.144528.

Practical Examples

IV

12

Challenges and Opportunities in Leading Systems Change

Jonathan Webb, Brian C. Castrucci,
Grace Castillo, and Kristina Y. Risley

CHAPTER OBJECTIVES

By the end of this section, the practitioner will be able to:

- Describe empirical examples of systems change leadership.
- Articulate common approaches to leading systems change.
- Engage in conversations with colleagues that help build a shared language about systems change leadership as well as an excitement to learn more or begin to implement the work.

INTRODUCTION

Systems change leadership involves working with diverse stakeholders to uncover the root causes of complex problems and identify fitting solutions. Some problems are simple and have easy fixes. Some challenges are complicated and can be addressed with the right expertise. Our most complex challenges, those we care deeply about in public health, are often complex and require significant inquiry to harvest a wide range of perspectives, alignment, coordination, and collaboration efforts and solutions. Using systems change leadership, we can see how actions we take within all levels of our systems—personal, interpersonal, organizational, cross-sector, political—create the systems, for better and worse, within which we live, work, play, and pray.

Sometimes our actions result in successes and serve as the foundation for further success and thriving communities. Sometimes our actions result in unanticipated short- and long-term problems that at best sustain the status quo and at worst cause damage to those in communities we had the best of intentions to help. In both cases, taking the time to understand cause-and-effect relationships lets us build on what we know works well. We also can grow a deeper understanding of the true nature of our problems—not just our perceptions of them—so that we identify solutions that are relevant and helpful; these solutions help communities thrive in the ways they want to thrive. Take, for example, a food desert: a simple, reasonable solution to lack of access to good-quality fresh food might be to open a food bank. This might or might not, however, be the right solution to an undefined issue. A systems change leader would take time to talk with diverse community members to find out what issues have caused the community to become a food desert. This process likely would yield a range of simple, complicated, and complex problems that could be addressed by individual community members and provide the opportunity for them to align and coordinate efforts as well as collaborate on new solutions to address explicitly identified issues of concern.

The types of complex challenges we face in our field are generally in the domain of what we call the social determinants of health—the conditions that keep health inequities in place no matter what solution we introduce. Diverse input from a range of community voices helps to ensure that we address the most relevant issues with effectual innovations. This moment in history, dominated by coronavirus disease 2019 (COVID-19) and heightened awareness of systemic and long-term racism, highlights the complexity of the circumstances that resulted in markedly poorer health outcomes for people of color. Racism is the foundational contributor to challenges faced by marginalized communities, including lack of access to high-quality education and unsafe homes and transportation. There is an urgency for systems change leadership that we have not seen in recent history. As public health practitioners, we are challenged to develop a deeper understanding of what is required for this type of leadership; the moment we're experiencing demands it. While obtaining these skills may be challenging, uncomfortable, and even daunting for some, it can also be exciting and rewarding, if we fully embrace the possibilities it may yield.

Systems change leadership is necessary work today and will continue to be critical work in the coming decades. Even as students graduate from schools of public health with deep scientific knowledge and strong public health technical skills, they will also need the leadership skills to effectively mobilize various types of partners, including community members who have expertise as a result of their lived experience. They will need to harness all of this understanding into actionable strategies to improve community and population health and especially the upstream factors affecting health—including the role of racism in keeping communities of color from achieving equitable outcomes.

This work involves more than identifying and bringing stakeholders together, something for which we in public health have a strong proclivity. It involves internal and external work to develop personal, interpersonal, team, and organizational and cross-sector leadership. It involves an intentional focus on introspection, the facilitation of honest conversations, consensus building, and sustainable action planning around a shared vision or agenda.

Systems change leadership lays the foundation for meaningful collaboration and increases the potential for improved understanding, efficiency, and actionable solutions. Most important, it raises the potential for equitable outcomes so that all people can achieve whole health. Following are two brief case studies of systems change leadership.

FEED THE CHILDREN

This example examines a promising attempt at systems change leadership in New Orleans' Lower Ninth Ward. Chapter author Jonathon Webb discusses his work in the following.

Background

This systems change leadership work took place in 2014 while I was a team lead for Feed the Children. Feed the Children focuses on international and domestic work around food insecurity. One of our domestic efforts centered on New Orleans' Lower Ninth Ward, 9.5 years after hurricane Katrina in 2005. In the simplest terms, our organization focused on addressing the problem of food insecurity within this neighborhood. We wanted not only to provide food resources to the community but also to address the environmental and systemic elements that created and perpetuated food insecurity, such as access to good-quality child care, jobs, and education.

Long before Katrina, there was abiding disinvestment in the Lower Ninth Ward. Prior to the hurricane, the Lower Ninth Ward could be characterized as a marginalized community that bordered New Orleans' French Quarter. After Katrina's devastation, the community was last in line to obtain recovery resources, even though the neighborhood had received extensive media coverage and photos of the community were circulated widely because of the ruinous impact of the storm. When our team began its work with the community, the neighborhood was by all definitions a food desert—it was hard for community members to buy good-quality food at a reasonable price. Community residents went to gas stations and small convenience stores for food; the nearest grocery store was several miles away.

We wanted to engage with and work alongside the Lower Ninth Ward's community, residents, and stakeholders in order to understand why there was food insecurity in the community and determine what we could do as partners to effect change. We wanted to provide food and address the underlying structural and systemic challenges that kept the community from thriving. One of the ideas that came up in our conversations with community members and stakeholders was to bring a grocery store to the neighborhood.

To stand up the store, we needed to work with a variety of partners. We were intent on working with community organizations, community leaders, and individual community members. Feed the Children would be the project's financial backer and it would also obtain funding from additional sources including local government, for-profit partners, and social venture capitalists. The goal was to partner with a local community grocery store operator who would run the store and hire individuals in the community, which would address the food-desert problem as well as bring jobs to local residents. We also planned to establish an onsite early childhood center, financially supported with grocery store proceeds. The goal, likewise, was to engage a team of community health workers from the community to help us understand the community's needs and to help connect them with healthier food options.

The suggested approaches addressed some of the root causes of food insecurity in the Lower Ninth Ward, including access to jobs and education. Addressing root causes would lessen the risk of families continuously experiencing food insecurity. Our inclusive, community-engaged process working with community stakeholders and members as well as community health workers would build community support for this project. Our efforts promised to bring food, jobs, early childhood education, and ultimately health to the community. Further, this work would tangibly support the community's desire to show that investing in communities like the Lower Ninth Ward was worthwhile and that many of the neighborhood challenges arose because of a historical lack of meaningful investment and not an inherent flaw in the community itself. The work would debunk long-standing myths and stereotypes about communities like the Lower Ninth Ward.

Nine months along, it appeared that all the necessary elements were aligned to carry out the project. Investors were engaged, funds were secured, and our team was working closely alongside the community. A grocery store owner was successfully selected and was willing to operate the new site; all of the pieces were falling into place. Unfortunately, in the end, the project failed because of an unanticipated land ownership issue. It was not possible to lay claim to a deed for the designated property because it did not meet the square footage requirements for developing a grocery store. In reality, the Lower Ninth Ward only had one property that met the budget and location criteria and had enough square footage to accommodate a grocery store. Sadly, the owner of this property passed away during the projected timeline for completion and as such it could not be purchased to support this project.

Lessons Learned

Although the project in the Lower Ninth Ward ultimately was not successful, we had a strong foundational approach and commitment to systems change, and there were many lessons learned that highlight important elements of systems change leadership.

Community-Driven Engagement Matters

The Feed the Children team prioritized community-driven engagement from the beginning. We wanted to work alongside the community and in concert with residents and stakeholders. We focused on working together to create a shared vision and priorities. We wanted a situation where the community wanted to work with us as much as we wanted to work with them. Through this process, the community saw us as a partner while they steered the ship; we were not the ship captain. Our team had resources and expertise to bring to the table, and the community had knowledge, lived experiences, community expertise, and other resources. In the end, we were the invited guests to this work even though we initiated the relationship; through the relationship design process described in the following, we talked through how we would work together to support the community.

Take Time to Build Genuine Relationships

Before we approached the community with the desire to address food insecurity in their neighborhood, the Feed the Children team had direct, honest conversations internally about how we should avoid going into the community with a paternalistic mindset that focused on what needed to happen in the community's best interest. Even though communities often accept help from organizations like ours, we knew that if we went into the community with an authoritarian "we know best" mindset, it would be impossible to build the trust needed to identify the core challenges in the community. Sustainable change would not be possible. Our team wanted to embrace the opportunity of partnership and co-creation of a shared vision, priorities, and sustainable action plan. To this end, our team applied its genuine relationship-building strengths to take the time to build relationships with community members, meet them where they were, learn what was important to them, and find ways that we could add value to addressing their needs.

This work was challenging and rewarding for me, our team, and our organization. As an African American male team lead who grew up in communities that looked like the Lower Ninth Ward, I had a level of understanding and comfort going into and working in similar places. We had shared experiences. At the same time, I did not want to assume that my experience growing up in urban Philadelphia was the same as those growing up in the Lower Ninth Ward. Nevertheless, because of similar upbringings we could find common ground, and this helped create trust in our relationships. Because the community trusted me, it helped residents also to trust the team, even though the rest of the team lacked shared experiences with the community.

NATIONAL CONSORTIUM FOR PUBLIC HEALTH WORKFORCE DEVELOPMENT

This example examines national systems change leadership efforts to support development and modernization of the U.S. governmental public health workforce. Chapter author Brian Castrucci participated in this work as president and CEO of the de Beaumont Foundation.

Background

The 1988 Institute of Medicine Report, *The Future of Public Health,*[1] called for broad, crosscutting skills and competencies for public health practitioners. In response, core competencies were developed for public health generally and for specific disciplines within the field (e.g., epidemiology, public health nursing, preparedness) or specific degree types (e.g., master of public health). This proliferation of competencies resulted in expansive lists of needed skills (from which it has been hard to discern priorities) and created a workforce of highly specialized and knowledgeable experts in distinct scientific disciplines such as epidemiology, laboratory sciences, chronic disease prevention, maternal and child health, environmental health, and injury and violence prevention. Competition among these specialty areas for legislative and public attention and categorical funding has nurtured silos rather than addressing the crosscutting needs common among public health workers.

While the scientific skills of each public health discipline are critical to delivering better health, the governmental public health workforce increasingly requires strategic skills including systems change leadership that allow workers to transcend traditional public health disciplines to meet the evolving needs of the public. The governmental public health workforce needs to bolster its programmatic and scientific capacities with a broader set of skills and knowledge that support the multi sector vision-setting and leadership needed to address the social, community-based, and economic determinants of health. A more integrative approach is needed to effectively manage initiatives, engage across sectors, and influence key factors that affect community health. The governmental public health workforce needs to develop strategic skills that complement its existing discipline-specific expertise with an ability to gain and apply knowledge from experts in other disciplines such as transportation, agriculture, and housing.

While many of these skills are not unique to public health, they are necessary to address the changing nature of the problems we face in public health. The problems we face today are complex and require input and understanding from a wide range of diverse stakeholders, development of shared visions, alignment around common goals and many solutions, and strategic implementation to avoid unnecessary duplication of effort. Development of these skills is necessary by those in our workforce if we intend to sustain and modernize governmental public health to ensure the health of our population.

In 2015, the National Consortium for Public Health Workforce Development, established by the de Beaumont Foundation, used a systems change leadership process that convened diverse public health stakeholders from more than 30 national public health membership associations, federal agencies, and public health workforce peer networks to identify areas of alignment among their workforce priorities. Based on a strong consensus, Consortium members urged prioritization of the development of strategic skills that complement the specialized skills and knowledge present in the governmental public health workforce. Through the Public Health Workforce Interests and Needs Survey (PH WINS), a partnership that includes the de Beaumont Foundation, the Association of State and Territorial Health Officials (ASTHO), the National Association of County and City Health Officials (NACCHO), and the Big Cities Health Coalition (BCHC), these strategic skills were confirmed by the public health workforce.[2] This national survey was a product of this systems change work that addressed a gap in our understanding about workforce interests and needs. It continues to provide longitudinal workforce data to understand the changing interests and needs of the governmental public health workforce.

The Consortium produced a report, "Building Skills for a More Strategic Public Health Workforce: A Call to Action (Consortium Report),"[3] that became a critical tool in advocating for national-level change in how we train our public health workforce. The call to action included: (a) elevate strategic skills to equal status with specialized skills, (b) invest in strategic skills development, (c) build systems rather than silos, (d) develop effective and engaging training, and (e) create a coordinating mechanism to make strategic skills a reality across the country. Updated strategic skills, necessary to address complex public health problems including racism, can be found in a new, 2021 de Beaumont Foundation report, "Adapting and Aligning Public Health Strategic Skills."[4]

Throughout the process of discussing and developing the original Consortium Report, we included leaders from our federal stakeholder group, including participants from the Health Resources and Services Administration (HRSA), which operates the national public health training center program. As a reflection of 30 different public health organizations, the thought leadership in the report became the foundation of a new direction for the public health training centers. Previously, HRSA trained practitioners in silos, such as preparedness center-specific funding. Because of the Consortium Report, HRSA began to focus on elevating the strategic skills identified in the report. HRSA's endorsement catalyzed the field to strengthen these crosscutting skills among public health practitioners. It also created momentum for increased focus on strategic skills more generally, including systems change leadership.

As important as this funding shift has been for workforce development, there is more to be done. Systems change leadership rarely has finite ends. The *process* did have a clear outcome: The immediate process outcome was that we modified tens of millions of dollars of federal funding. That is real. Nonetheless, the *change* will not have that same defined ending. We continue to work to influence training systems and health departments to adopt this ideology. We want these strategic skills to be integrated into curricula in schools of public health and into professional development opportunities for practitioners.

We also sought to engage in systems change leadership by creating the coordinating mechanism described in the 2017 report. To this end, in 2019, the de Beaumont Foundation engaged a revitalized National Consortium for Public Health Workforce Development that includes some of the original Consortium members as well as new participants, all of whom are critical public health workforce stakeholders, to mobilize around a common agenda for public health workforce development.[5] With an eye on equity through the selection process, stakeholders include national, state, and local public health workforce experts. To date, a founding committee—that helped shape the process to identify and align workforce stakeholders including the creation of a Consortium steering committee—and the steering committee have engaged in significant work to understand the root problems related to public health workforce development and create a vision and mission, guiding principles, roles and responsibilities, and workforce focus areas and goals. These focus areas and goals were vetted with individuals at all levels of the workforce, making it a top-down, bottom-up, and all-around process to ensure collective buy-in and identify the best opportunities to change how we support and develop the public health workforce. As the National Consortium continues to apply this collective impact approach in its ongoing work, the proposed solutions could spread and bolster the wider workforce for decades to come.

This work is being used to leverage change at multiple levels, including with the Biden administration's commitment to workforce development. There is an urgency around workforce development that has never existed before, making this work particularly timely. Health disparities have worsened and received increased attention because of COVID-19. Our increased awareness of racism as a public health problem is amplified by the Centers for Disease Control and Prevention's recent declaration of racism as a public health problem and the need to build the capacity of the public health workforce to lead systemic change to make substantive advancements in the equitable care of people of color.

This work has the potential to leverage real change related to public health workforce development because those leading it took the time to engage diverse stakeholders, build relationships, and move together toward a common workforce development vision. They were committed to stopping and regrouping when things were about to go off-track. Acknowledging individual and collective input, celebrating small and large wins every step of the way, and being transparent and clear in communications about the process have heartened all those involved in this work at all levels of participation.

Lessons Learned

Stakeholder Engagement

It was critical to bring diverse stakeholders to the table and to align around and identify workforce needs, garner support for the strategic skills approach to workforce development, and advocate for funding efforts to support workforce development through a strategic skills lens. It was important to be inclusive in our approach to engage a wide range of stakeholders. It gave critical players the opportunity to have a voice, even if it was an unpopular voice or seemed to be a detractor—often, such a voice indirectly addressed an unspoken need or want. Further, a systems change leadership approach allowed all stakeholders to share risk as well as celebrate successes together; the whole is always greater than the sum of its parts.

Persistence and Long-Term Commitment

The people behind thought leadership and reports aim to effect change at the systems level. The Consortium report "Building Skills for a More Strategic Public Health Workforce: A Call to Action" led to immediate, long-lasting changes in funding structures, which in turn changed how we train and develop the public health workforce.[3] We must maintain support for that change, and we are working to make sure we can continue to evolve the field. The Consortium continues its commitment to creating a coordinating mechanism for all stakeholders to align and act on a wide range of public health workforce priorities and activities. Primary focus areas include health equity in the workforce and the work completed by the workforce, public health pipeline and recruitment, and ongoing learning and professional development. Making incremental shifts in the public health workforce is a long game—systems change leadership takes time. Celebrating small victories along the way provides the necessary commitment to stay with the journey.

Resources

We do not always see or have the time and resources to explore underlying root challenges, and as a result, we focus on solutions to unclear problems. Focusing on root challenges is how we begin to engage in systems change leadership. Large-scale systems change requires investment of time and other resources. It is important to appreciate the time, resources, talent, and treasure that it takes to bring about these changes.

Short-term funding may limit organizations to focusing on immediate, tangible problems rather than deeper, systemic challenges. Funders need to see results, which can lead organizations to be cautious and focus on clear-cut, winning issues. It is important for funders to understand that systems change is about a process as well as outcomes. It takes time to get desired results from systems change leadership work. Making headway on this issue requires a strong business sense and a commitment to being excellent stewards of resources.

Timing

Some systems change issues are so complex that it can be easy to stall while analyzing the root problem rather than chipping away at the problem itself. Practitioners must consider timing. What is the right balance between moving too quickly—essentially, wasting time, energy, and credibility by not being thoughtful—and moving so slowly that the initiative does not get under way?

In addition, particularly for work in racial and health equity that incorporates community-engagement components, progress must happen at the speed of trust.[6] Public health practitioners can come into a community well-intentioned and ready to move forward, but if a team has not spent the time to build confidence with those in the community who may or may not trust outside groups, progress will stall. Many communities and residents have very real experiences of being taken advantage of or exploited. When an organization comes into a community, it is a mistake to push through without taking the time to build trust with individuals.

Workforce Development

The public health workforce has always been one of the field's greatest assets. A strong workforce is essential in systems change leadership. Give newer and more seasoned staff the opportunity to grow and develop into systems change leaders. When given the opportunity, encouragement, and support, staff will be creative and innovative. Our public health practitioners devote time, talent, and treasure to work in our field to improve community and public health; they could work in other places that are not committed to the greater good. We do not want our practitioners to come into public health and then burn out because of constraints they experience related to fighting bureaucracy to get things done. We also need to build a pipeline of systems change leaders and realize that today's leadership may not look or act like leaders in the past. These factors must be considered in recruitment and benefit packages. With the proper support, training, and learning opportunities, practitioners in the field will have the necessary skills to lead, speak, and create systemic change.

CHAPTER SUMMARY

This chapter painted a vision for the type of change that is possible when we focus on systems, including the integration of policies and practices that result in shifts in culture that help lead to the creation of vibrant, adaptable, and thriving communities ranging from a neighborhood to a public health workforce. Today's world challenges us to change fast, do more with less, and do everything in a context of constant stress. In undertaking systems change leadership work, we must expand our mindset by listening and truly hearing our partners, change cultures, dismantle old and malfunctioning systems, and build new systems that allow all people to thrive. This work is not easy, but it is necessary and rewarding, especially when our goal of equitable systems that create the conditions for all people to thrive is clear and in the forefront of our efforts.

This chapter reviewed examples of systems change successes and challenges, exploring both a national systems change effort related to development of the public health workforce and a community-based systems change effort focused on food insecurity in New Orleans. Those people leading these systems change efforts applied skills that have the potential to make significant headway in the long-standing systemic challenges we face in public health. While there always will be critics of systems change leadership, commitment to developing these skills and the rewards they yield in the form of changed systems that are equitable are worth it.

Surround yourself with people who support systems change work. Create the conditions for sustainable change by developing genuine, ongoing, and long-term relationships with your stakeholders. Commit to the public health long game while celebrating small successes along the way. Work with our current reality, COVID-19 and heightened awareness of systemic racism, to generate the urgency needed to engage others in systems change. This is a critical time, when we have the opportunity to make a 180° turn in our business-as-usual approach to public health. Do not let the moment pass you by.

Key Messages

- **Be bold.** If you think you are already thinking bold, think even bolder. That is the heart of systems change. As part of being bold, look outside usual partners, especially from a funding perspective. As hard as it is, practitioners cannot be afraid of failure. For every good report that catalyzes systems change, there are a thousand that do nothing. Embrace the end goal. What are you trying to do? What do you need to fix? Then, work it backward.
- **Have honest conversations.** Be honest with impacted community members, with yourself, and in your organizations. Commit to understanding why and how you reached the current situation, no matter what problem you are trying to solve. For example, people of color historically have been intentionally forced to sit out. As the country was being designed and developed and systems established, people of color were set to the side and disenfranchised, then eventually

invited into the conversation *after* the rules were set. If we are honest in our conversations, we can be bold in our solutions.

- **Check your ego.** Sometimes honest conversations hurt. We must develop the skills to check our egos at the door so we can listen earnestly and truly understand a challenge and how to approach it. Another component of looking beyond ourselves is understanding that we may not be the person who ultimately needs to solve a problem—it is always a group effort. Sometimes we lead and sometimes we follow; strong followership is also a form of strong leadership.

- **Prioritize effective, genuine community engagement.** One aspect of genuine community engagement is engaging meaningfully with community members. This may require some training, because not everyone comes naturally to this skill set. Practitioners must be able to converse with community members to expand partnership opportunities rather than contract or shut them down. Create a concrete strategic plan for the partnership that sets realistic expectations and milestones. This gives people a sense of what every stakeholder can bring to the table, what gaps need to be filled, the scheduled timeline, and how community members can most effectively engage. If an organization is truly partnering, it should be following and working alongside communities. Collaborative planning is the foundation for genuine community engagement.

Tips

- **Recognize scope.** The scope of systems change matters. Changes at the town, county, and state levels are all different from one another. When you try to change the field, expect it to be hard—there are many disparate, moving parts.

- **Be clear.** Bring stakeholders together and then clearly identify the problem in plain language. Stay away from jargon.

- **Identify interests.** It is essential that all stakeholders have a clear understanding of what they stand to gain from being at the table. Many people are motivated by self-interest, so ensure that everyone knows why they are there. Once you have identified others' interests, include additional people who are not natural partners.

- **Appreciate the limits of consensus.** Change is hard; systemic change is harder. You will not please all of the people all of the time. Make sure you have engaged diverse stakeholders, listened to them, and then acted to the best of your ability given the data. You do not need to act on all stakeholder input, but it is important to understand all perspectives so that you make the best decisions moving forward. See all people, hear all voices.

- **Understand your position.** Different organizations have different advantages. Foundations are not beholden to a government agency. Funders can say different things than government agencies can.

REFERENCES

1. The Institute of Medicine (IOM). *The Future of Public Health*. National Academy Press; 1988.
2. de Beaumont Foundation. Public Health Workforce Interests and Needs Survey. https://debeaumont.org/wp-content/uploads/2019/04/PH-WINS-2017.pdf. Published 2019.
3. de Beaumont Foundation. Building Skills for a More Strategic Public Health Workforce: A Call to Action. https://debeaumont.org/news/2017/building-skills-for-a-more-strategic-health-workforce-a-call-to-action. Published July 18, 2017.
4. de Beaumont Foundation. Adapting and Aligning Public Health Strategic Skills. https://debeaumont.org/strategic-skills. Published March 2021.
5. de Beaumont Foundation. A Common Agenda for Public Health Workforce Development. https://debeaumont.org/phworkforcesurvey. Published 2021.
6. Covey SMR, Covey SR. *Speed of Trust: The One Thing That Changes Everything*. Free Press; 2018.

13

Public Health Systems Change in Action: Transforming Organizations Toward New Strategic Directions

Jeannine Herrick and Ray Dlugolecki

CHAPTER OBJECTIVES

By the end of this chapter, the practitioner will be able to:

* Describe systems-thinking frameworks that public health practitioners can apply to practice.
* Apply practical techniques for advancing systems strengthening within an organization.
* Connect concepts related to systems thinking to real-world examples.
* Articulate the importance of relationships in systems thinking efforts.

INTRODUCTION

This chapter provides an overview of systems change efforts in state and local governmental public health agencies.

THE NECESSARY SHIFT TO SYSTEMS CHANGE IN GOVERNMENTAL PUBLIC HEALTH

As a field, public health has a growing, common understanding that the way our work is currently funded and structured will continue to produce inequitable health outcomes unless we intentionally engage in the dismantling of current systems and the structures that support them and rebuild in new ways. The focus of many public health agencies is centered on transactional programs and services that feel necessary, even lifesaving. When we step back and take the big-picture view, continuing to invest most of our limited resources in downstream efforts will lessen our ability to solve the root causes of complex problems. This chapter outlines some examples and practical approaches to shift a portion of our resources toward strategic efforts to change systems. These resources might include financial, human, and political capital. Systems thinking and tools provide an opportunity to examine existing systems and structures to determine which need adapting versus which need dismantling and rebuilding. Using systems thinking tools reveals leverage points to help guide decisions about where to focus efforts to yield high-impact results.

Systems change work is still change work, and to be successful it should follow best practices in change management. This should start with understanding and communicating that change is a process that happens over a sustained period. Shifting toward systems change work is not an add-on initiative; it is a transformative, inside-out experience. It takes considerable effort in the beginning stages to explain why a shift is important in such a way that it resonates and the benefits become clear for the people served, the staff, and the organization overall. Stakeholders and staff need multiple opportunities to be introduced to the reasons for the change.

Systems change work begins with asking ourselves, "How well do we understand the systems that affect health for the various populations that we serve?" As people start to experiment with the idea of describing and doing their work differently, they should be supported with training, mentoring, or other supports to build confidence.

This chapter gives real-life examples of public health organizations that have engaged with systems change efforts with multi-sector partners at different levels. The first example highlights how Florida's internal change management work happened in parallel with the design and implementation of systems change interventions. Following this are four short examples of local governmental public health agencies that each went through an internal change process to create new functional capacities. Lastly, this chapter presents an in-depth example of a local health department in Jackson County, Missouri, that was focused on one central concept: Health depends on more than just a visit with a healthcare provider—it is the product of countless interrelated factors.

PUBLIC HEALTH SYSTEMS CHANGE AT THE STATE LEVEL: FLORIDA

In 2017, Florida's Office of Children's Medical Services Managed Care Plan and Specialty Programs (CMS), the state's Title V Children with Special Health Care Needs (CSHCN) Program, sent a team to the National Maternal Child Health Workforce Development Center with a desire to improve the way they were serving children up to age 21 and their families. The goal was to increase treatment among children with a behavioral or mental health condition, as almost half of Floridian children in need of mental health services were going without, according to the National Survey of Children's Health and National Outcome Measure 18.

They were particularly interested in piloting and scaling an integrated model across the state that would bring pediatric primary care and behavioral health together. Their vision was to center the experience of families and work with community and state partners to create a seamless, culturally appropriate service delivery system catering to the needs of individual children. The challenge was in how they would strategically collaborate, implement, and provide sustained support to the intricate web of partners at state, regional, and local levels.

The behavioral health integration work was a prelude to a broader transformation of the agency's CSHCN work. Florida's CMS leadership planned and then announced that they would enhance their Managed Care Plan functions, which included case management, by contracting with a vendor. Strategic investments in workforce development ensured that staff who wanted to continue in case management could successfully move to the vendor agency.

A second team then took advantage of the Workforce Development Center's development and coaching. They created a regional hub model to bridge community system supports broadly and tied to Title V CSHCN priorities, with a focus on access and quality. This shift would task staff to lead population health initiatives with partners and strengthen systems to better serve the CSHCN population, using a regional hub model.

With a focus on transformation of their remaining workforce to oversight and strategist-related roles and functions, training and supports were provided for the staff who stayed to develop systems thinking–oriented capacities. These included building multi-sector relationships and networks, facilitating the growth of referral networks, and executing new roles for family leaders.

When strategic leadership is tied to meaningful purpose it will retain the staff needed to roll out the implementation. They learned to listen, adapt, and co-create. They arrived at wholly new conceptions of what their work was, who would do it, and how the system would support the work (including expanding the role for family leaders inside the system from direct service to population health opportunities). And they discovered that learning how to use systems change tools is different from developing a systems thinking mindset; the workforce shift to a new mindset is crucial and requires utilizing team members in various new capacities, encouraging creative ideas, and making space for dissent as part of the change management process. Lastly, they didn't just build their own capacity. They helped their partners build capacity, new relationships, and new network capacity in the process.

Florida's ability to see the big picture and critically analyze the larger system that CSHCN and its families navigate helped them identify where components needed redesigning. The shift from technical, service delivery work to systems integration and prevention-focused population health was tremendous in three ways: the effort to build workforce capacity, the courage to push for bold system improvements, and the benefits CSHCN and its families are experiencing. Lessons learned that could be applied in other contexts include: (a) Take a big-picture perspective and ensure that all streams of work are aligned with the strategic questions your organization is committed to addressing: Look for where downstream approaches have gotten away from organizational purpose. (b) Advocate for bold system improvements: Use multiple communication strategies to explain why the change warrants buy-in throughout the organization. (c) Early in the process, consider the implications on staff and what the potential workforce capacity needs will be to support the change effort.

PUBLIC HEALTH SYSTEMS CHANGE IN LOCAL GOVERNMENTAL PUBLIC HEALTH

The Kresge Foundation sponsored the Emerging Leaders in Public Health program that developed approximately 100 leaders from local governmental public health agencies. These leaders applied strategic leadership skills and competencies toward building capacity within their agencies to assume reimagined roles that will be transformative for their local communities. Below are four examples of how local public health leaders can use systems change concepts and tools to inspire new ways of thinking that help agency staff and partner organizations focus on the strategic questions that will move the dial on stubborn, hard-to-solve health inequities.

For years, the state of Oklahoma had the distinction of incarcerating women at the highest rate across the world. The Oklahoma City-County Health Department (OCCHD) recognized that public health could play a role in reducing that rate, especially among African American women. OCCHD saw this as part of their overall work integrating public health practices with social services, including education, criminal justice, primary care, and mental health. They did a deep dive into gathering information from various points across the criminal justice sector and learned that collective resources with partners should first be invested in an improved data-mapping strategy. Later, they were able to advance a component of their original goals; OCCHD embedded community health workers within the Oklahoma County Drug Court system to work with residents being released from incarceration, providing health and social service supports and thereby disrupting re-entry cycles. This work was greatly facilitated by the trust established through new partnership building and the data system–mapping work.

Lessons learned that can be applied to other beginning systems change work include: (a) Identify and interview as many as possible of the key stakeholders about how they view the problem and potential solutions: Physically leave your office and make the effort to visit others in their environment. (b) Bring authentic curiosity and the desire to learn more to the process: Welcome uncertainty of where the work will go beyond the first few steps. (c) Approach new relationships with a spirit of generosity: Consider what you might be able to offer as opposed to advancing the interests of your well-intentioned agenda.

The DuPage Heath Department in Illinois recognized that mental health emergencies were distressing the local emergency departments, paramedic response teams, and the police force. Furthermore, residents in crisis were not receiving the specialized care they needed. Related, the local jail was unable to meet the growing mental health needs of its incarcerated population. Through extensive community partner building, the DuPage Health Department created a role for their agency to serve as a bridge between both the mental health and criminal justice systems. Together with community partners, they participated in a Sequential Intercept Mapping workshop that allowed them to see the whole system and all its interconnecting components, which facilitated setting a broad collective agenda. From that agenda emerged a multitude of system improvements that have continued to evolve and multiply. These improvements have included creating a trained mobile mental health post-crisis response team, hiring a former probation officer as a re-entry specialist to work with soon-to-be-released inmates, and reducing nonclinical admissions to local emergency departments by offering a mobile crisis response program for police departments.

Most persistent problems that affect population health are complex, so taking time and effort to understand the big picture of a system, and acknowledging its complexity, is a good starting point for collective work with partners. Using a trained facilitator who can encourage generative discussion to elicit a common understanding of the subcomponents of the larger system and then visually reflect to the group the drivers and outcomes can help the group identify the key leverage points to zone in on and how to prioritize them. The leaders in DuPage knew they couldn't do everything at once, so they were selective about where to begin. As they built success in one area, the benefits were felt across the whole system and then they could confidently move on to the next.

The Las Animas-Huerfano Counties Health Department in southern Colorado sought to improve the health and well-being of their youngest population in the hopes that it would disrupt cycles of intergenerational poverty and stress. They achieved their first goal of integrating primary care, community partners, and behavioral health with a seamless referral process for CSHCN. Through the extensive process of seeking community perspectives, they began to understand the system dynamics and limitations that were affecting children's ability to thrive, including lack of access to high-quality early education and early assessment and treatment for behavioral health, which resulted in more school-age children struggling with academics and overall social–emotional development. In response, they became involved in both local and state policy efforts and helped advance the Colorado Behavioral Health Task Force and legislation for universal Kindergarten and Pre-K. They expanded their efforts to build the advocacy skills of local partners to influence state policies that were affecting their ability to best provide comprehensive, accessible, holistic services to children.

Their extensive listening sessions with residents and partners helped them design a village approach, leading to building a campus offering comprehensive services with a "warm hand-off approach." This method integrated trauma-informed best practices into multiple sectors within the larger system to improve children's health and well-being in their context. While these problems are not uncommon in many contexts, the leaders in Las Animas-Huerfano were unique in their approach. As others approach similar population-based challenges, some actionable steps include (a) Hold deep and intensive listening sessions with community-based partners: Ask questions to staff at varying levels and do not limit your inquiries to leadership only. (b) Be brave and advocate for legislation changes if they are a key driver in the challenges you hope to address: You do not need a law degree to influence policy change. (c) Go beyond building your own capacity in something transformative like policy change: Work to build other groups' capabilities as well through training, coaching, and mentoring.

In Minnesota, Saint Paul-Ramsey County Public Health's leadership recognized that there are many possible applications for systems level improvements with cross-sector partners to collectively shift power dynamics that have historically disproportionately benefited White families. To influence the overall system over time as they applied their agency's new role as the prevention strategist for well-being and health, they began by building a partnership with social services and the impacted community to co-create a transformed child welfare system. The collective goal was to reduce racial bias in the removal of children from their families and those that love them into the foster care system. Both agencies have learned and made improvements to this system, and the public health department has expanded its focus to explore an array of applications of the prevention strategist role. This new role for the agency is directly reflected in their strategic plan, and efforts are underway to build internal capacity to lead multiple community efforts from a systems perspective. Lessons learned from leadership in St. Paul include: (a) Co-creation is slow and sometimes feels hard, be patient. (b) Choosing one specific aspect of a larger system to build success is a great way to get started. (c) Public health leaders assuming leadership roles within cross-sector partner agencies and vice versa can help build momentum for overall systems change efforts that span institutional boundaries.

LOCAL SYSTEMS CHANGE CASE STUDY: JACKSON COUNTY HEALTH DEPARTMENT

One of the authors, Ray Dlugolecki, assistant director of public health, along with the health director, Bridgette Shaffer, helped lead an organizational role transformation within the Jackson County Health Department. Our agency is a mid-sized health department serving approximately 380,000 residents just outside of Kansas City, Missouri, across urban, suburban, and rural communities. Our agency is one of the few health departments in the nation that is managed and operated by a healthcare system—the largest safety net system within the Kansas City region. In recent years, our agency has intentionally focused on building and supporting community to make meaningful progress on addressing deeply rooted community health issues.

As a health department, we recognized that our health challenges were often tied to upstream drivers and contextual factors that are interconnected, but our programs and services were largely focused downstream. Across the landscape of our community partners, there exists no single "hero" within the web of cross-sector partners who could solve all our problems. Instead, it was clear that we needed to work together to examine these health issues in different ways and design new solutions that would better address upstream drivers.

Agency leadership came to the realization that our own organization needed to shift internally before we created a new role identity within the community. We were selected to participate in the ELPH program, which provides leadership and organizational supports to local health departments to create a new agency role. Our initial desire to become the Social Determinant Resource Navigator for the healthcare system in Jackson County was borne out of the need to ensure that healthcare providers could better identify patients' needs based on their social determinants. We would then provide an easy-to-navigate referral system for patients to access appropriate, interconnected resources.

At the start of this journey, we thought that we had a solid grasp on the most significant challenges facing our community and which programs and solutions would create the most meaningful impacts. Only after using systems thinking tools such as causal loop diagrams and network mapping with community groups did we recognize that there were deeper issues related to the community-wide array of systems of programs and services that would require a different approach to be effective. We learned that collaborative solutions without strategic insights do not result in truly adaptive work that can effectively address upstream drivers. For example, in our community, the unintended consequences of fragmentation among service providers addressing the opioid crisis perpetuated the status quo, despite the investment of resources. Too often in the region, investment was reactionary, without any thought as to how the dynamics between service organizations contributed to the challenge. These insights led to calls for reform among how organizations strategized about the opioid crisis, and for a more collective approach focusing on high leverage points.

In our collaborative work sessions on equity with community partners, we used systems thinking tools. Through that process, we learned about the challenges facing specific populations in accessing institutionalized programs and services. We were surprised to learn about the layers of complexity that affect community members' ability to access healthcare, such as reimbursement and payment structures, early childhood disparities and inequities, provider cultural competency, segregation by income and race, and many other factors. While health insurance remains the primary discussion point, the complexities and inequities in accessing healthcare will require a strategic restructuring of the whole system. Otherwise, we will not make meaningful headway on improving access to care. These tools, along with facilitation guides for generative discussions, provided us with a new perspective from which to see potential combinations of approaches and solutions across institutions that could begin to redefine entrenched systems that were producing our current results.

We realized that our work and the work of our partners often overlooked the broader system at play, moving toward overly narrow and overly simplistic interventions that may produce some of the desired effect without changing the overall system. Our interventions were often transactional, helping individuals negotiate existing structures for short-term gain but leaving the existing structure in place.

The goal was to implement a portfolio of solutions that were transformational, such as policy initiatives that cross multiple institutions, moving efforts toward proactive solutions. These types of solutions alter the ways institutions operate, thereby shifting cultural values and political will to create equity and change systems. In the context of homelessness, a transactional solution might be creating a homeless shelter—necessary, but operating within existing structures. A transformational approach to homelessness could be implementing policy solutions that guarantee affordable housing for all, decreasing economic inequity, or creating universal access to healthcare. Applying transactional fixes in silos perpetuates a lack of connection across organizations and groups working to improve community health, creates misalignment among efforts, and contributes to inequity and gaps in service.

From this realization, we set forth to become a "community integrator" agency within Jackson County—the go-to for systems thinking and analysis within our local public health ecosystem. In short, we, with our partners, wanted to get better at challenging the massive underlying issues that drive so much of our residents' health outcomes. Our goal was to define a new operating model for public health—one in which we thrive at the systems level and are truly able to influence systems in a strategic and direct manner.

INTERNAL TRANSFORMATION—PEELING BACK THE LAYERS

Public health operates within complicated systems and subsystems all relating to the health of a community. Through our journey to understand this complexity with more clarity, we looked for leverage points where collaborative solutions could begin to shift the drivers or root causes of health inequities.

Health systems are comprised of the formal health system, complex social systems and dynamics surrounding specific groups of people, and economic and political systems of opportunity and power. Each of these subsystems has another layer of subsystems within them. The formal healthcare system has both curative health and preventive health systems. Because of the interconnectedness of these systems, it is impossible for any single organization to claim that they alone can solve population health challenges.

Through listening sessions and deep discussions with community partners and residents, we came to understand that if we hope to challenge these large, underlying issues that drive so many of the challenges that we see in our community, collectively we must improve our ability to assess and understand persistent problems related to population health and integrate our interventions across institutions.

Community health lacks the role of integrators—people, teams, or organizations that have a dedicated function to work across subsystems to help create a positive outcome at the end. In order to make a difference on problems and complex issues such as health disparities, racial equity, and economic mobility, we need a workforce that can work across various subsystems.

The starting point for us and our partners, we realized, was to step back and reflect on the big picture of how these pieces could be aligned toward a strategic direction. A system or structure is set up to do exactly what it is currently doing. In our community, and across the nation, the healthcare system perpetuates inequity and segregation by income and race because of how financial benefits and reimbursement are structured. Yet we often fail to name this for what it is when discussing access to care. This system is doing exactly what it is designed to do—it is not inherently evil. There is a collective acceptance that took place across our community partners. Although our collective intentions were to ensure Black, Indigenous, and People of Color (BIPOC) populations were experiencing equitable access to healthcare, in reality the overall system was set up to continually sustain conditions that contribute to poor health outcomes. We had to acknowledge this difference between intention and reality and then work together to determine what portfolio of coordinated interventions could change the conditions. We learned that true improvements may require change or the complete decimation and rebuilding of system structures.

RATIONALE FOR AN ORGANIZATIONAL SHIFT

Our team began by making alterations to our health department's mission, vision, and values. We had always valued equity, but as we learned more about the systems supporting health inequities, we came to realize that valuing equity was going to have to mean something different going forward. The exploration of our organization's values guided our revised mission and vision. As we started to imagine our new vision for the future, it became apparent that we were going to need to dismantle some existing systems that were not serving our residents, especially our BIPOC residents, and replace them with newly designed systems. We could see that our original hunch to connect services across the community in a more seamless way was going to be important, as would be shifting the focus of those services to be substantially more prevention focused. Because ensuring the health and well-being of a community that has many different populations living within is complex, we hoped that a focus on systems would provide the boost to impact we desired.

RESTRUCTURE

We altered several of our agency positions to facilitate this organization-wide role transformation. We altered our primary data analyst job description from functioning as a traditional data/epidemiologist to focus on network analysis and building capacity for systems dynamics modeling and agent-based modeling. These capacities are useful to visualize and explain how complex system structures are designed. They provided analytical tools to aid us and our partners in making sense of complexity. Our new staff member helped colleagues learn the basic applications of systems change by providing analytical support during decision-making. As we take partners through a process of creating a causal loop diagram or a stock-and-flow diagram, we wanted to understand how changes in inputs impacted the overall system.

LEADERSHIP DEVELOPMENT

Leadership development in adaptive thinking and systems thinking is immensely helpful to lead systems change efforts. Two senior leaders led the role transformation work while participating in an applied learning-focused leadership development program. An expanded leadership team participated in subsequent capacity building in the concepts, skills, and applications of systems tools, equity approaches, change management, and communication.

STAFF DEVELOPMENT

We needed to ensure our staff had a safe space to participate in difficult conversations that are necessary to challenge system structures. Staff needed to feel comfortable asking questions about why their jobs were changing, why the way we approach serving our community was changing, and what this means on both a personal and organizational level.

We were intentional to ensure that systems thinking skills were integrated across the organization. Everyone had ownership of and commitment to this new way of working, including policy staff, health educators, and all staff with community interfacing roles.

Over time, we have worked to develop critical thinking skills and analytics capacities among all staff so that they can facilitate and participate in conversations that can lead to positive systems change. At a minimum, we hope that all staff can see the bigger picture of an overall system with systems components within and ask meaningful "what if" questions that stimulate meaningful exchange of ideas with partners, stakeholders, and community members.

We worked with our staff to embrace the concept of complex collaboration, which we see as involving both the close examination of systems components and drivers and the identification of the leverage points that will have the greatest impact for coordinated intervention across partnerships. For example, we now prioritize an examination of the network of stakeholders and community members who are at the table to work on complex community challenges before we determine our strategies or initiatives. Doing this ensures we have the right people at the table to thoroughly perform a systems analysis and understand the complexities and dynamics among all parties involved in the work.

The most significant part of agency role creation and staff development efforts was around our enhanced organizational focus on equity. As an agency, this is our ultimate "why," the reason behind the role change at its core. We wanted to make sure that we were intentionally incorporating equity concepts into our interactions with each other and the community members we serve. We wanted equity to be at the center of our design of programs and services. We dug deep into systems thinking to understand the power dynamics around drivers of poor health outcomes, with the intention of finding the right mix of interventions to shift those power dynamics for more equitable outcomes. We worked with an expert consultant group to facilitate engaging conversations with staff about personal bias and bias within systems and productive, supportive ways to work together toward common goals related to equity. Leadership received additional supports so they could model and provide guidance to staff as they engaged more deeply in equity work. This body of work was a process, which took place over a sustained period.

TOOLS

From our internal work and preparation came new tools at our disposal. These tools would eventually support the new functions of our agency.

Five Rs Framework

The five Rs framework was our initial introduction to the notion that many frameworks for health behavior change and policy change may be entirely too simplistic without explicit inclusion of systems components from the beginning to the end of the program life cycle. The five key dimensions—results, roles, relationships, rules, and resources—provide methods to understand the layers and surrounding context of an existing system. This framework provides structure for cultivating a systems practice across a team, organization, or institution. The framework helps collective groups see complexities within and across systems, analyze various components and subcomponents for additional clarity, and then develop coordinated approaches that are designed to change systems.

Causal Loop Diagramming

The health department trained staff to use causal loop diagramming as a tool in their work, and now our whole agency decided to use it as part of our larger community health assessment and improvement processes. Using a systems approach in our agency's overall assessment and planning will be a change for staff who work on direct services or specific programs or services. Part of shifting to a systems change perspective as an agency is to help staff see the value in redesigning the structures of our organization so that they align in intentional ways with community partners to address the drivers of our most persistent health inequities.

Causal loop diagrams help to visualize how different variables in a system interconnect and influence its behavior. It is a visual way to tell a story of how a collaborative group imagines a system is working and contemplates what might shift the behaviors of the system. Causal loop diagrams articulate how certain variables or drivers can increase or decrease a potential focal variable. Linking loops that emerge can tell a story. Reinforced loops indicate where an intervention may have a big impact.

Causal loop diagrams can be as simple or complicated as you like. The four basic elements include variables (drivers), the links between them, the indication on a link to show how variables are interconnected, and the indication on a loop to show what type of a behavior the system will produce. For example, if I'm interested in learning more about the rate of substance use of an adolescent population, the driver of self-image has a link. As self-image is more positive (+), substance abuse decreases (–), showing an opposite relationship.

In group-facilitated sessions, it is always interesting to see what loops emerge and how similar or different they were compared to what assumptions group members held about how a system was functioning. Most interesting is doing multiple causal loop diagrams for the same system but for different populations or contexts. This is critically important when working to center equity, as the emerging loops and relationship dynamics may be vastly different, demonstrating that the same system improvements efforts will not work equitably for everyone. Causal loop diagrams indicate where the leverage points are in a system.

Network Mapping/Network Analysis

Network analysis is a helpful way for collaborative efforts to gain common understanding of the interdependence among systems players. They can identify strengths or weaknesses in relationships, levels of connectedness, levels of trust, and to what degree a system is cohesive or fragmented. There are many possible uses for network mapping in community-based population health work. We used network mapping to identify and understand the organizations that were working on the opioid crisis. This exercise revealed the array of services and providers, showing where strategic relationship facilitation could improve efficiency and effectiveness. Staff at our agency used a free, publicly available application, kumu.io, to create visually appealing and interactive network maps of systems we were working within. This resource has been included at the end of this chapter.

SYSTEMS WORK CULMINATION—ConnectHERE

We were so passionate about this new systems work within our agency that we branded it ConnectHERE, with a mission to serve as a community integrator—using systems thinking to advance transformative solutions that improve health for all people. ConnectHERE is both an initiative of the health department and a community lab for systems thinking and experimentation. Our long-term goal is not only to create a space for health department staff to lead work on systems, but also to build capacity for other community partners to recognize the importance of systems in their own work. ConnectHERE functions to consolidate important tools to improve public health's ability to assess, understand, and build systems (Exhibit 13.1).

EXTERNAL APPLICATIONS

One of the initial projects of ConnectHERE was creating an integrated referral system (IRIS) for organizations to refer clients across non traditional partnerships based on

---

EXHIBIT 13.1 ConnectHERE Guiding Principles

- *Collaborative Innovation*—Recognizing that no one organization or person has all the solutions.
- *Organizational Equity*—Equity must be integrated in organizational culture in order to practice it at the systems level.
- *Experimentation*—Recognizing that we, with the community, have the ability and duty to design our future and our systems, not just make tweaks to previously designed systems.
- *Playing at the Systems Level*—The complex health challenges we face will require the coordination of people and solutions across industries, sectors, beliefs, political ideologies, and disciplines currently existing in silos.

their social needs. As partners refer people from organization to organization based on their needs, the health department gets valuable data and insights on the safety net system in Jackson County. These data are dependent upon the robustness of the network of organizations participating, but over time we will learn of safety net systems gaps, misalignments in services, and inefficiencies. From these data and our focus on the systemic structure overall, we can make recommendations that inform a collaborative approach for improvement, such as identifying organizations that are not actively involved in the social safety net system but may be addressing the underlying root causes of challenges facing our community.

It is imperative that these organizations are brought into the collaborative processes to document the dynamics of the system around particular challenges. In addition to specific projects, ConnectHERE is building frameworks and toolkits to use in facilitation efforts with organizations and community networks through a defined five-step community process to ensure systems thinking and strengthening is at the forefront of collaboration. The first step in this community process is *design*. In this step, we list all the functions that are necessary throughout the systems to produce good health for everyone. That is, we design a system that we, with our partners and the community, imagine would work perfectly. Then, we *map* the overall system to determine how all the different pieces would need to work together to function perfectly. The third step is to *analyze*. For the sake of paving a path forward, we pick out and analyze the parts of the system that do not seem to be functioning perfectly to assess all our possible options for intervening. Fourth, we *model*. Since we will likely have many potential interventions but limited resources, we model all our options to create the greatest possible impact. Finally, we *act* by choosing the highest impact interventions to comprise our portfolio and implement them with ongoing monitoring, evaluation, and learning.

Broadly speaking, we work with community partners and residents to design ideal systems in the beginning of the exercise. This way, we ensure the historical constructs do not interfere with communities' abilities to imagine the future. Next, we explore ideal system functions against current structures, analyzing bottlenecks and areas for improvement. This allows us to model selected interventions that will ultimately contribute to a portfolio of high-impact solutions that can be implemented in a collaborative manner. While it sounds simplistic, the process needs to be framed in a safe container for difficult conversations and opportunities for innovation. We ask our partners and residents to challenge the status quo, which is often difficult when discussing systems that have been perpetuated for generations. We believe that this collaborative process will ensure our interventions are rooted in strategy, providing results framed in efficiency and effectiveness.

FUTURE ITERATION

Future phases for our network efforts include expanding and improving referral options and creating a more well-rounded image of the system. We hope to have multiple rounds of network analysis on referral data to provide to stakeholders with insights on system functioning. We hope to implement social determinants of health screening for partners. We are striving to produce network resiliency reports for various communities to inform strategy.

Future phases of our external application work will apply lessons learned from one community within our county to expanded work in neighboring communities. We hope to adapt the initial agent-based and system dynamics models to a web-based application for stakeholder use. We are looking to create a portfolio of interventions for integration into the model. Eventually, we would like to add applications to the website that would allow stakeholders to test a portfolio of solutions to improve systems dynamics.

Lastly, we hope to launch a consulting arm for ConnectHERE to help community organizations and other public health agencies use systems and network analysis tools to further their strategic efforts.

CHAPTER SUMMARY

To challenge and change the underlying drivers of poor health outcomes, we need to develop capacity around analyzing, understanding, and building systems. Three main groups of systems operate and interact to influence health outcomes: the formal health system, complex social systems and related dynamics, and economic and political systems of opportunity and power.

To shift from a current state that lacks clarity related to an equitable, functioning community health system to a future state that has a portfolio of interventions to transform a community health system toward equitable, sustainable, and positive results, a five-step process is helpful to frame the transformation. Steps for this process include: (a) design, (b) map, (c) analyze, (d) model, and (e) act.

Relationships with stakeholders including staff are key for the success of any change effort; this is especially true for systems change. Shifting to systems change perspectives can lead to new roles for organizations and requires intentional leadership and workforce development supports.

Building capacity in systems thinking is a process, as it is a different way of thinking. With time and practice, everyone can develop systems thinking capabilities.

Systems change work should always be co-created with partners. Systems are interconnected and systems change often requires dismantling something existing. Different organizations have different terminology, collaborative norms, and stakeholders and priorities. Investing time and effort into going slow and building trust is key for any systems change effort to be successful.

Key Messages

- In order to move away from transactional interventions that provide only short-term gain we need to consider how collective efforts could proactively change the *broader system* surrounding persistent population health challenges.

- Complex collaboration and coordinated interventions take time, trust, and a willingness across partnerships to dismantle something existing before putting changes in place. Go slow and build in lots of opportunity for *relationship building, reflection, and iteration.*
- Shifting power dynamics that contribute to inequities requires the right mix of coordinated interventions. There is considerable trial and error so test before scaling up and intentionally build in *opportunities for learning.*

Tips

- Taking time and effort to understand the big picture of a system and acknowledging its complexity are good starting points with partners. Systems thinking tools and highly skilled facilitation can help.
- Build leadership and staff capacity in adaptive and systems thinking to participate in conversations that can lead to positive systems change.
- Visiting tours to partner organizations and extensive listening sessions with community members can jumpstart collaborative work and ensure that systems solutions are designed in ways that will truly benefit those they intend to serve.

Supplemental Resources

- Kumu—website for organizing complex data into relationship maps: kumu.io
- Systems Integration Resources/Systems Integration Core at the National MCH Workforce Development Center: https://mchwdc.unc.edu/areas-of-focus/
- Time to Transform: Adaptive Approaches for Population Health. Northwest Center for Public Health Practice. Public Health Institute. 2020: www.nwcphp .org/training/time-to-transform
- ReThink Health: A Rippel Initiative: www.rethinkhealth.org/about/
- Systems for Action: http://systemsforaction.org/
- Aligning Systems for Health (Robert Wood Johnson Foundation/Georgia Health Policy Center): www.alignforhealth.org/aligning-systems-for-health/
- Dawn of Systems Leadership: https://ssir.org/articles/entry/the_dawn_of_system _leadership
- Senge PM. *The Fifth Discipline: The Art & Practice of the Learning Organization* .Crown; 2010: https://books.google.com/books/about/The_Fifth_Discipline .html?id=b0XHUvs_iBkC

BIBLIOGRAPHY

Peters DH. The application of systems thinking in health: Why use systems thinking? *Health Res Policy Sys.* 2014;12(51). Accessed March 26, 2021. http://www.health-policy -systems.com/content/12/1/51.

Sacks E, Morrow M, Story WT, et al. Beyond the building blocks: Integrating community roles into health systems frameworks to achieve health for all. *BMJ Global Health*. 2019;3:e001384. doi:10.1136/bmjgh-2018-001384.

Senge PM. *The Fifth Discipline: The Art & Practice of The Learning Organization*. Crown; 2010. Accessed March 26, 2021. https://books.google.com/books/about/The_Fifth _Discipline.html?id=b0XHUvs_iBkC.

Senge P, Hamilton H, Kania J. The dawn of system leadership. *Stanf Soc Innov Rev*. 2015;13(1):27–33. doi:10.48558/YTE7-XT62.

The 5Rs Framework In The Program Cycle. Updated October 19, 2020. Accessed March 26, 2021. https://usaidlearninglab.org/sites/default/files/resource/files/5rs_techncial_note_ver _2_1_final.pdf.

14

Community Leadership: Collaborative Leadership in Action

Dorothy Cilenti and Lacy Fehrenbach

CHAPTER OBJECTIVES

By the end of this chapter, the practitioner will:

- Learn about community change frameworks and practices.
- Learn the fundamental skills of successful systems change efforts at the community level.
- Be able to increase awareness of community change efforts that are achieving results in one state.
- Learn systems change tools to apply in public health practice that address the root causes of inequitable health outcomes.

INTRODUCTION

In previous chapters, we learned about leadership at the personal, interpersonal, team, and organizational levels. This chapter explores leadership at the systems level and public health's role as health strategist for guiding community change to improve health. Community-level change results when those most impacted by social challenges have a say in designing and implementing solutions. The participation of intended beneficiaries and their families, neighbors, and trusted leaders can be an integral part of community health strategies to achieve better results. We touch on the importance of building relationships and working within and across sectors on an ongoing basis and not just when a problem arises. We highlight that communities are not problems to be solved but opportunities waiting to happen.

FRAMEWORKS AND PRACTICES

Factors that impact health are much broader than whether someone has access to healthcare when they are sick. Education, income, quality of housing, and safety of neighborhoods influence how long and how well we live. For some, ingredients for a healthy life are readily available; for others, particularly those who are Black, Indigenous, People of Color (BIPOC), or People with Disabilities, the opportunities for health and well-being are significantly limited. Health equity, or the idea that everyone, regardless of race, ethnicity, gender, income, location, or any other factor, has a fair and just opportunity to be as healthy as possible, must drive what we do at the community and systems level. A framework called Public Health 3.0 was released in 2016 and lays out five recommendations for governmental public health agencies to meet the health challenges of the 21st century.[1] The first recommendation is that public health leaders must assume the role of health strategist for the communities they serve. This role requires engaging multiple sectors and working with all stakeholders to address the social determinants of health. The Robert Wood Johnson Foundation (RWJF) Culture of Health Action Framework identifies priorities organized under distinct action areas for driving measurable, sustainable progress and improving the health and well-being of all people. A culture of health is broadly defined as one in which good health and well-being flourish across geographic, demographic, and social sectors; fostering healthy equitable communities guides public and private decision-making; and everyone has the opportunity to make choices that lead to healthy lifestyles. Leading toward a culture of health requires making health a shared value for everyone, fostering cross-sector collaboration; creating healthier, more equitable communities; and strengthening integration of health services and systems to achieve improved population health, well-being, and equity.[2] This framework is useful in thinking about how health strategists may achieve better health through creating a culture of health in their communities.

EXAMPLES OF COLLABORATIVE LEADERSHIP PRACTICES IN ACTION

It Takes a Village to Go Back to School

In March 2020, Washington state ordered all public and private K–12 schools closed as a community mitigation intervention to slow the spread of coronavirus disease (COVID-19). Because of the uncertainty of the new and evolving pandemic, schools remained closed through the end of the school year. As the summer and fall approached, work began to navigate a path forward for a gradual return to in-person learning during the pandemic.

While the governor can use emergency powers to close schools statewide, local education administrators are ultimately responsible for establishing appropriate education services. Because COVID-19 is a public health emergency, the local health officer should be involved in advising their schools, but the local school board, superintendent, and principal play lead roles in making decisions about the return to in-person learning.

The decision to return to in-person learning is among the most complex and challenging any community could face. Schools are fundamental to child and adolescent development and well-being. In-person learning has a broad range of benefits for children and adolescents. In addition to educational instruction, schools support the development of social and emotional skills; create a safe environment for learning; address nutritional and behavioral health and other special needs; and facilitate physical activity.[3] The absence of in-person learning may be particularly harmful for children living in poverty, children of color, English language learners, children with diagnosed disabilities, and young children, and can further widen inequities in our society.[4]

While schools are generally among the safest and most supportive environments for children, they are congregant settings. During a pandemic, it is imperative to return to school in a way that balances these well-known benefits with the risks for transmission within the school, which places at risk the health of students; staff; the families they return home to, which may have adults who are vulnerable to severe disease; and the broader communities in which they live.

Despite many plans, exercises, and recommendations for how to close schools, a playbook for returning to classrooms during a pandemic did not exist. In addition, the science of COVID-19 and the effect of its exposure on children was just starting to emerge and there was little information available regarding how the reopening of schools could impact disease rates and transmission in the surrounding community. This left many states and communities on their own to figure out if and for whom they should provide in-person learning, how to start, and how to stay open once they did.

Interests and positions related to reopening schools are diverse and juxtaposed. There are the staff and administrators of the school—these are the people who make schools so great for our children and communities. Some of these staff or members of their household may be at risk of severe COVID-19. There are the children and their families. Within families, there is great diversity of needs, capacities, preferences, concerns, and personal situations. Employers in the community have workforces that rely on schools to care for their children during much of the workday.

Health and Safety Guidance

As the first wave of COVID-19 subsided in Washington state, the Washington Department of Health (DOH) began developing guidance about how to provide in-person learning in schools that chose to do so. Staff reviewed the protocols of other countries that resumed schools, the guidance for similar sectors like childcare, the science on respiratory viruses, and the emerging science around face coverings and COVID. With funding from the DOH, the University of Washington regularly produced a "LitRep," or literature report, on key topics, including school reopening, which was instrumental to decision-making.

The Office of the Superintendent of Public Instruction (OSPI), the state's education agency, convened a health and safety workgroup that consisted of superintendents, principals, and labor union representatives. The DOH brought suggested guidance to this group. The DOH also connected with other states, local public health, and the Centers for Disease Control and Prevention (CDC). In early June 2020, Washington state was among the first states to put out K–12 Health and Safety Guidance. The protocols in this guidance were required of any public or private K–12 school under a Governor's Proclamation related to COVID-19. The guidance required: daily symptom monitoring, face coverings for all students and staff, 6 feet of physical distance in most instances, frequent handwashing/sanitizing, increased cleaning, improved ventilation and air quality, and cohorting (assembling small consistent groups) of students where possible. It also required local school and public health officials to be prepared to respond to cases and potential outbreaks with timely diagnostic testing, contact tracing, and isolation and quarantine.

At the time the guidance was released, very few states or local jurisdictions were requiring face coverings among adults, and only a few required it of children or students. It was extraordinarily controversial. Letters poured in on the subject, primarily in opposition. People were skeptical children would wear them. Some worried it was dangerous physically or psychologically for children to wear masks. Over the summer, DOH leaders went on a webinar tour to talk through the science behind the guidance and tips for implementing it. They sought earned media wherever possible to talk about mask wearing, including tips for parents and caregivers about how to help children become comfortable wearing masks. Washington state ran a broader statewide masking campaign and put a Secretary's Order in place that mandated the wearing of face coverings in all indoor public spaces and outdoors whenever within 6 feet of others. In parallel, the evidence supporting mask use grew, the CDC and national groups like the American Academy of Pediatrics recommended mask use, and several other states mandated the use of masks in schools. Since June 2020, the DOH has continued to monitor the science and provide updated guidance. Evolving science has consistently supported the importance of strong disease mitigation measures as foundational for a safer return to in-person learning. However, several months into the school year, there were still concerns among some families and staff. The state met regularly with healthcare providers, local public health representatives, school administrators, educators and school staff, and the statewide parent–teacher association and provided these groups science reviews to help spread facts through the most trusted messengers.

In addition, to help ensure the safety of school employees, the DOH and OSPI worked with the state's Department of Labor and Industries to provide guidance around the appropriate types of personal protective equipment (PPE) for key scenarios and staff in schools. Many school districts went in together to bulk purchase PPE in the summer of the 2020–2021 school year, and the state maintained an operational reserve of PPE for healthcare providers, first responders, and key frontline workers like childcare centers and schools, in case there were supply chain issues over the course of the year.

Metrics to Guide Decision-Making

As disease levels rose in July 2020, more school staff and families began to question if it was safe to return to school. After consultation with several local communities struggling with decisions about whether to return and who should be prioritized, the DOH and a workgroup of local public health officers began developing metrics to guide local decisions about whether to begin, expand, or reduce in-person instruction for public and private K–12 schools during the COVID-19 pandemic. Again, staff turned to the experience and data from other countries that had resumed some level of in-person learning. These countries generally had low and decreasing community rates of cases of COVID-19. The incidence rates in several countries that successfully resumed in-person instruction were below 50 cases per 100,000 population per 2 weeks.[5]

In addition to having lower and decreasing community rates of disease, these countries took a cautious approach to resuming in-person instruction. Most countries first resumed in-person instruction for a portion of their students, and many implemented health and safety measures like physical distancing, frequent handwashing, use of face coverings, and frequent cleaning to reduce the spread of COVID-19 in the schools.[6]

Based on this information, a study from the Institute for Disease Modeling,[7] and engagement with key stakeholders, the DOH released advisory metrics and recommendations based on community case rates, with defined ranges for high, medium, and low. The DOH also recommended that schools consider test positivity and trends in cases and hospitalizations, as well as the broader risks and benefits to children and their families as they made decisions. The DOH favored a cautious, phased-in approach to resuming in-person instruction, starting with younger students, with additional students attending in-person school over time. They also noted the need to ensure the schools were prepared to implement all the health and safety measures and that the school and local public health agency were prepared to respond quickly to cases with testing and contact tracing.

A handful of other states released metrics around the same time. Washington's were fairly similar to other West Coast states, and generally cautious (Table 14.1). The CDC released metrics several weeks later. In Washington state, the majority of public school districts were where most of Washington's 1.1 million public school students spent the fall learning remotely. According to data from the OSPI and the Association of Educational Service Districts (AESD), as of October 2020, 91% of Washington public school students lived in districts that were providing some level of in-person learning. However, in most districts, in-person learning was limited to small group instruction of the youngest elementary students or students with special needs. Over the

TABLE 14.1 Washington State Department of Health Recommendations Regarding the Provision of In-Person Learning for K-12 Students Released Within the Decision Tree August 2020

COVID-19 CASES PER 100,000 OVER 2 WEEKS	RECOMMENDATION IN BRIEF
>75	Distance learning with option for in-person learning in small groups for students with highest needs and youngest learners
25–75	Phase in elementary then middle school in-person learning
<25	Provide in-person learning for all students

fall, letters poured in, this time primarily from parents and caregivers, worried about the impacts distance learning had on their children.

Schools that opened in Washington and across the nation, including at higher disease rates, provided more data around the risks of COVID-19 being introduced in schools and impact of health and safety measures on transmission. In Washington state, outbreak data showed that, while cases and outbreaks do occur in schools, recognition of transmission of COVID-19 has been limited in the school setting. There were 84 outbreaks between August 1 and December 12, 2020. A total of 266 cases are linked to these 84 outbreaks. The number of school outbreaks was larger in counties with higher community transmission; however, the size of outbreaks is, on average, small even in areas with high disease levels. Half of the outbreaks in K–12 schools had three or fewer cases linked. Seventeen outbreaks were larger, with five to 11 cases linked.

In addition, models from the Institute for Disease Modeling (IDM) suggested that the risk of transmission in K–12 schools depends on the incidence of COVID-19 infections in the community as well as school-based countermeasures.[7] A follow-up report from the IDM found that risks could be significantly mitigated through hybrid school schedules or via a phased-in approach that brings back K–5 first.[8] A third modeling study found that *when R effective is already at 1* in the surrounding community (meaning, disease levels are stable and not increasing or each person who has COVID-19, on average, infects one other person), reopening schools would not significantly increase community-wide transmission, provided sufficient school-based interventions are implemented, such as masking, physical distancing, and screening students and staff for symptoms. The use of hybrid scheduling further reduced the infection rate.[9]

Based on the early experience in Washington, additional science, and modeling studies, public health leaders in Washington state began consideration of broader ranges that would expand access to in-person learning at higher case rates. They looked at other states' metrics, as well as the CDC's and Harvard Global Health's Pandemic Resilient Schools guidance. Conversations with leaders were complex and difficult as cases, hospitalizations, and deaths were rising sharply in Washington state and across the nation. The state, under Governor Inslee's leadership, put severe restrictions in place, temporarily closing indoor dining, fitness, and similar sectors to avoid overwhelming the healthcare system. Communication was key—state and local public health leaders had to help people understand that schools needed time to plan. Releasing the metrics in December 2020 allowed them to plan for a quarter/semester break in late January or early February. With input from public health officials, stakeholders, and the governor's and state superintendent's leadership, Washington state ultimately decided on the metrics in Table 14.2.[10] Many stakeholders supported and embraced the change, and several districts began phasing in in-person learning in January and February. Educators and school staff, especially in western Washington, remained concerned though.

Testing

To further support return to in-person learning, the DOH in partnership with local health officials, school administrators, and school nurses developed school testing

TABLE 14.2 Washington State Department of Health Recommendations Regarding the Provision of In-Person Learning for K-12 Students as Updated Into a Toolkit for Decision-Making December 2020

FOR WHOM SHOULD YOUR COMMUNITY PROVIDE IN-PERSON LEARNING? GUIDELINES FOR SCHOOL ADMINISTRATORS, LOCAL HEALTH OFFICERS, AND COMMUNITY STAKEHOLDERS

The risk of COVID-19 being introduced into the school and spreading depends on the health and safety measures taken by schools and the level of COVID-19 spread in the community. **Consider the following educational modalities based on community transmission and other health and education risks and benefits.**

	HIGH	MODERATE	LOW
COVID-19 activity	**>350 cases/100K/14 days** Test positivity >10% Trends in cases and hospitalizations	**Approx. 50–350 cases/100K/14 days** Test positivity 5%–10% Trends in cases and hospitalizations	**<50 cases/100K/14 days** Test positivity <5% Trends in cases and hospitalizations
Education modality	**Phase in in-person learning in groups of 15 or fewer students for pre-K through grade 5 and those with highest needs** Prioritize pre-K through grade 3, students with disabilities, students living homeless, or those farthest from educational justice. If schools can demonstrate the ability to limit transmission in the school environment, add grades 4–5	**Phase in in-person learning prioritizing elementary (pre-K–5) if they are not already receiving in-person learning, and middle school** If schools can demonstrate the ability to limit transmission in the school environment, add high school when case rates are below about 200/100K/14 days	**Provide in-person learning for all students**
Extra curricular activities	Cancel or postpone most in-person extra curricular activities except those allowed under Safe Start and Governor's proclamations on COVID-19	Extra curricular activities must follow K–12, applicable Safe Start protocols and Governor's proclamations on COVID-19	Extra curricular activities must follow K–12, applicable Safe Start protocols and Governor's proclamations on COVID-19

(continued)

TABLE 14.2 Washington State Department of Health Recommendations Regarding the Provision of In-Person Learning for K–12 Students as Updated Into a Toolkit for Decision-Making December 2020 (*continued*)

FOR WHOM SHOULD YOUR COMMUNITY PROVIDE IN-PERSON LEARNING? GUIDELINES FOR SCHOOL ADMINISTRATORS, LOCAL HEALTH OFFICERS, AND COMMUNITY STAKEHOLDERS

Transition	**Across all COVID-19 Activity Levels:** ■ When trends in cases and hospitalizations are flat or decreasing, and the school can demonstrate the ability to limit transmission in the school environment, expand access to in-person learning. ■ When trends are increasing, pause expansion of additional in-person learning and maintain access to in-person learning for those who have it. Schools are not required to reduce in-person learning or revert to remote learning based on metrics if the school can demonstrate the ability to limit transmission in the school environment. ■ Consider other health and education risks and benefits to children and their families. At any COVID-19 level, transition temporarily to full distance learning for 14 days when school meets criteria in the Department of Health's K–12 Health and Safety Guidance or on recommendation of the local health officer.

guidance to help local school and public health leaders make determinations on who, how, and when to test students and staff in the K–12 school environment. This guidance then informed a pilot supported by a partnership among the DOH, the Gates Foundation, and the participating school districts and their local health jurisdictions.

The goal of this pilot was in-person learning and schools staying open once students have returned. In addition, Washington aimed to determine the costs and benefits of each approach, and if and how the state could scale from 13 districts in the pilot to statewide. The DOH with support from partners in philanthropy and the private sector also created a "Learn to Return" playbook that gave schools step-by-step guidance on how to carry out testing, regardless of which approach they are using; reporting; and basic contact tracing. The playbook also included communication tools for families and staff, example forms, and decision tools. The first phase of the pilot included 13 school districts representing 120,000 public school students (approximately 10% of Washington's public school children). The second phase expanded to more than 70 districts. The program included three types of testing:

■ Diagnostic testing of people who have symptoms or are close contacts or cohort members of a case
■ Diagnostic testing plus repeat testing of asymptomatic staff
■ Diagnostic testing plus repeat testing or surveillance testing of asymptomatic students

The rapid diagnostic testing was critical for responding to and mitigating outbreaks as well as increasing access to low-barrier community-based testing for students, staff, and their families. Both benefits helped schools remain open after students returned to in-person learning. Repeat testing built confidence among staff or families of students and provided some surveillance data regarding COVID-19 in schools. Early lessons learned from the pilot suggested that testing can support returning to learn on a clear path to re-opening, but the effectiveness of testing services when school staff is hesitant for return to in-person learning still needs to be determined. In addition, the capacity to administer the tests was the most significant challenge—it needed to be easy for schools and local public health providers, both of which were already stretched. To date, demand for repeat testing for students has been limited, though this could change as more districts return and as more older students begin in-person instruction, and with the release of the CDC's Operational Strategy for K–12 Schools through Phased Mitigation. The DOH explored a few partnerships with end-to-end providers of testing support in the pilot in hopes of finding a good mix that made testing easy for schools and local public health providers, and accessible for students, staff, their families, and the broader community. The DOH also engaged the Health Commons Project, a local non-profit, to help run the program and support schools. As school testing continues to expand, it is the state's hope that schools, which often serve as a service hub in the community, can provide an access point to COVID-19 testing for the broader community as well.

Vaccine

The COVID-19 vaccine was an additional tool in the toolbox to help with a return to in-person school. To inform Washington's allocation of the limited supply of vaccine, the DOH used their state's data on COVID-19 cases, outbreaks, hospitalizations, and deaths; the National Academies of Science, Engineering, and Medicine's framework for Equitable Allocation of the Vaccine for the Novel Coronavirus; the recommendations of the Advisory Committee on Immunization Practices; and broad stakeholder engagement. The DOH conducted 90 interviews and focus groups with 568 people across the state and received 18,000 responses to a survey available in multiple languages. Key groups include African American/Black communities, Latinx communities, Pacific Islander communities, immigrant and refugee communities, older adults, people experiencing homelessness, farmworkers, people with underlying health conditions, and individuals with disabilities. Communities and sectors at higher risk for getting or spreading COVID-19 were also intentionally engaged. This included essential workers and businesses, healthcare workers and providers, college students, youth, education and early-learning providers, and parents. In commitment-to-Washington's Government-to-Government relationship with Tribal Nations, Tribal Nations and American Indian/Alaska Native communities were also engaged. The results of their engagement are summarized in COVID-19 Vaccine Prioritization Guidance and Allocation Framework (available online at www.doh.wa.gov/Portals/1/Documents/1600/coronavirus/820-112-InterimVaccineAllocationPrioritization.pdf). Ultimately, the allocation framework in Washington centered on the goal to reduce severe morbidity and mortality and the negative societal impacts resulting from the transmission of SARS-CoV-2. To develop the COVID-19 Vaccine Prioritization Guidance and Allocation Framework, they emphasized proactive community engagement, transparency, evidence, and fairness.

Within this framework, school staff who provide healthcare services were eligible in Phase 1A, and any person in Washington 65 years or older was eligible in Phase 1B Tier 1. Most school staff fell into Phase 1B in Tiers 2 (for those aged 50 or older who are at higher risk for severe morbidity or death) and 4 (for all others). School staff were recognized and prioritized as critical frontline workers and because lack of in-person learning leads to a negative societal impact. While school staff were near the front of the line for vaccines, supplies were limited in Washington state and nationwide. Neighboring states put school staff on parallel track to the elderly, whereas people 65 and older were prioritized in Phase 1B Tier 1 in Washington. In early March 2021, President Biden announced that all K–12 and childcare staff were immediately eligible. Washington public health leaders had been planning vaccine administration partnerships to get these workers protected and sped up these plans by about 2 weeks.

Spring Developments

In March 2021, while most districts had begun returning to in-person learning, there were still a few without plans to return that school year. In addition, preliminary data suggested relative increases in emergency department visits for suicidal ideation, suspected suicide attempt, and psychological distress, and pediatricians reported seeing significant increases in youth with eating disorders, anxiety, mood disorders, and depression with suicidal thoughts or self-harm behaviors. The governor declared a Children and Youth Mental Health Crisis. Among other things, this proclamation directed all schools and districts to provide an option or some in-person learning by April 5 (elementary school) or April 19 (middle or high school). The mental and behavioral health impacts, combined with additional science supporting that layered prevention and mitigation measures limit transmission of COVID-19 in schools even when community transmission is high, led to the sunsetting of the state's K–12 metrics and decision tools. Schools must provide an in-person option for learning (hybrid is acceptable). Families continue to have a fully remote learning option.

In March, the CDC and DOH relaxed physical distancing requirements based on emerging science and studies from schools that had used less than 6 feet or at least 3 feet of physical distance in schools.

The DOH began publishing a monthly report on outbreaks in schools and has been carrying out more detailed interviews among schools with outbreaks to better understand which layered prevention and mitigation measures help limit transmission in schools. This informed the following school year's guidance.

Final Thoughts

As of March 15, 2021, 58% of elementary students and 51% of all grades were receiving at least some in-person instruction weekly. Some communities in Washington returned to in-person learning with the Health and Safety Guidance. Others needed guidance and metrics or testing. Some communities required guidance, metrics, testing, and vaccinations before families and staff had the confidence to return. Starting in April 2021, all schools had to provide some in-person instruction. Whatever these communities needed, Washington public health and education leaders were ready to adapt and innovate to meet the unique local needs. The state was already looking toward the 2021–2022 school year to anticipate needs for updated guidance, mental health, and social supports for students and staff, and other needs for stronger and more resilient K–12 schools and pandemic recovery.

APPLICATION TO PRACTICE

Erwin and Brownson describe five critical capacities and capabilities needed by the public health workforce in order to carry out the role of health strategist, including systems thinking, communication skills, the willingness to work outside of traditional comfort zones in an entrepreneurial fashion, transformational ethics, and policy analysis and response.[11] In the Washington state example, systems tools enabled leaders to understand, plan, implement, and evaluate changes at the systems level and across all sectors and partners that needed to work together to address these challenges. Start with a systems approach by applying systems tools early and often. Tools such as asset mapping and causal loop diagramming can be found at www.mchnavigator.org/trainings/systems-integration.php.[12]

Leaders must also be competent in strategic communication, which means defining the target audience, developing the correct message, and using this information to select the appropriate communication channels or messengers. Given the dynamic situation with science emerging throughout the pandemic, the level of distrust of governmental communications, and access to an enormous amount of inaccurate information via social media, the public health workforce in its role as health strategist must master the art of translating research into practice and policy. Public health and education leaders in Washington state conducted webinars about mask wearing in the case example, including tips for parents and caregivers about how to help children become comfortable wearing masks. Washington state also ran a broader statewide masking campaign. The state also met regularly with healthcare providers, local public health and school administrators, labor, and the statewide parent–teacher association. For additional communications resources for public health practitioners, visit the Public Health Communications Collaborative website at https://publichealthcollaborative.org/.

Moreover, leading with an entrepreneurial orientation means leaders must be proactive, innovative, and willing to take risks. Risk taking may be challenging within governmental public health but has been a key element of success in other sectors, such as business. In some cases, it means being willing to be first or move early, as Washington did in requiring its health and safety measures such as face coverings and physical distancing. In others, it means being willing to adapt and be flexible as Washington was with metrics and testing.

Creating partnerships with the private sector to facilitate implementation of innovative approaches to improve community health is an important component of an entrepreneurial orientation. In the case example, public health leaders in Washington state schools supported school districts in their efforts to bulk purchase PPE in the summer for the 2020–2021 school year, and the state maintains an operational reserve of PPE for healthcare providers, first responders, and key frontline workers such as childcare providers and school personnel in case there are supply chain issues over the course of the year. The DOH forged partnerships with COVID-19 testing services to help address workforce gaps and make the provision of testing easier for schools and local public health. The Superintendent of Public Instruction forged a partnership with a major healthcare system to vaccinate school staff when eligible in the state's framework. The DOH and local public health worked to ensure access to vaccination among school staff outside of that provider's service area. Think about ways that public health goals may align with those of the private sector. For tools to explore innovation, check out the Public Health Innovation Playbook at www.phnciplaybook.com/.[13] Here you will find an interactive website and resources to help you set the stage, identify the problem, generate ideas, and pilot and implement your ideas.

In addition, it is not sufficient for the health strategist to improve overall population health, as this improvement may also worsen health inequities by providing advantages to certain populations and further hurting those most in need. For example, recent research shows that the establishment of new parks in historically marginalized neighborhoods can result in housing price increases and the displacement of low-income people of color.[14] Thus, public health leaders in their role as health strategist must ensure that whatever health improvements are made for the public overall must be made equally for all communities. The vaccination allocation framework in Washington, as we learned in the case example, centered on the goal to reduce severe morbidity and mortality and negative societal impact due to the transmission of SARS-CoV-2 but also prioritized ethical principles of maximum benefit, equal concern, and mitigation of health inequities. School staff in Washington state were prioritized among the first group of frontline critical workers in congregant settings, which also included childcare, agricultural, food processing, correctional facility, and law enforcement workers. Find resources to help you center equity in your decision-making with the Racial Equity Alliance's Racial Equity Toolkit, available online.[15]

Lastly, one of the most important skills for the public health leader as health strategist is to identify and analyze policy changes and their impact on community health. Public health leaders in Washington state recognized that the policy to close schools during the COVID-19 pandemic created an absence of in-person learning that would likely widen inequities in the state and be particularly harmful for children living in poverty, children of color, English language learners, children with diagnosed disabilities, and young children. Identifying policy changes and responding effectively and appropriately must be a well-honed skill of the health strategist. To learn more about building skills in policy analysis and policy making, go to www.cdc.gov/policy/analysis/process/index.html for a practical guide to the CDC's process.

CHALLENGES AND OPPORTUNITIES

Though the concept of a health strategist is new, a focus on social determinants of health and health equity in public health is not. However, challenges such as limited funding and bureaucratic inflexibility create barriers to meaningful, sustained community health improvement. There are some examples, though, like those described earlier, of leaders on the front lines adapting, innovating, and transforming health. They are not doing this alone, however. They have learned the importance of engaging others in this work, particularly those with lived experiences. To get started, talk with diverse stakeholders, including community members, and ask them about what would work to create health equity and improve the well-being of all.

CHAPTER SUMMARY

In this chapter, we described how the COVID-19 pandemic is an unprecedented and rapidly changing time for public health leaders who must effectively partner with a broad range of stakeholders across multiple sectors to address the social determinants of health. As demonstrated through the example, we can work through the response to intentionally forge partnerships and change systems to support longer-term goals and work that improve health equity and social justice. Shared accountability to ensure the conditions in which everyone can be healthy regardless of race, ethnicity, gender identity, sexual orientation, geography, or income is necessary to create and sustain safe and thriving communities. These challenging times demand collaborative leadership that centers equity and leverages strategic alliances to improve population health.

Key Messages

- Public health leaders must assume the role of health strategist for the communities they serve. This role requires engaging multiple sectors and working with all stakeholders to address the social determinants of health.
- Systems tools enable leaders to understand, plan, implement, and evaluate changes at the systems level and across all sectors and partners that need to work together to address these challenges.
- Public health leaders must master the art of translating science into practice and policy.
- Identifying policy changes that may negatively impact the health and well-being of marginalized communities and responding effectively and appropriately must be a well-honed skill of the health strategist.

Tips

- Anticipate needs for health literacy, mental health, and social supports for communities disproportionately impacted by poor health outcomes.
- Adapt and innovate to meet unique needs of communities.
- Be proactive and willing to take risks.
- Engage others in this work, particularly those with lived experiences.

Supplemental Resources

- National MCH Workforce Development Center: https://mchwdc.unc.edu
- Robert Wood Johnson Foundation Align for Health: https://alignforhealth.org
- Building Leadership—Community Tool Box: https://ctb.ku.edu
  building-leadership
- National Implementation Research Network: https://nirn.fpg.unc.edu/
  national-implementation-research-network

REFERENCES

1. DeSalvo KB, Wang YC, Harris A, Auerbach J, Koo D, O'Carroll P. Public health 3.0: a call to action for public health to meet the challenges of the 21st century. *Prev Chronic Dis.* 2017;14:170017. doi:10.5888/pcd14.170017.

2. Trujillo MD, Plough A. Building a culture of health: a new framework and measures for health and health care in America. *Soc Sci Med.* 2016;165:206–213. doi:10.1016/j .socscimed.2016.06.043.

3. The importance of reopening America's schools this fall. Centers for Disease Control and Prevention website. https://www.cdc.gov/coronavirus/2019-ncov/community/schools -childcare/reopening-schools.html. Accessed August 1, 2020.

4. Levinson M, Cevik M, Lipsitch M. Reopening primary schools during the pandemic. *New Eng J Med.* 2020;383:981–985. doi:10.1056/NEJMms2024920.

5. Michaud J, Kates J. What do we know about children and coronavirus transmission? Kaiser Family Foundation website. https://www.kff.org/coronavirus-covid-19/issue-brief/what -do-we-know-about-children-and-coronavirus-transmission/. Published July 29, 2020. Accessed August 2, 2020.

6. Guthrie BL, Tordoff DM, Meisner J, et al. Summary of school re-opening models and implementation approaches during the COVID 19 pandemic. https://globalhealth .washington.edu/sites/default/files/COVID-19%20Schools%20Summary%20%28updated %29.pdf. Published July 6, 2020.

7. Schools are not islands: We must mitigate community transmission to reopen schools. Institute for Disease Modeling. https://covid.idmod.org/data/Schools_are_not_islands_we _must_mitigate_community_transmission_to_reopen_schools.pdf. Accessed November 29, 2020.

8. Maximizing education while minimizing risk: Priorities and pitfalls for reducing risks in schools. Institute for Disease Modeling. https://covid.idmod.org/data/Maximizing_ education_while_minimizing_COVID_risk.pdf. Accessed November 29, 2020.

9. Testing the waters: Is it time to go back to school? Institute for Disease Modeling. https://covid.idmod.org/data/Testing_the_waters_time_to_go_back_to_school.pdf. Accessed November 29, 2020.

10. Washington Department of Health. Tools to Prepare for Provision of In-Person Learning among K-12 Schools. https://www.doh.wa.gov/Portals/1/Documents/1600/coronavirus/ DecisionTree-K12schools.pdf. Accessed March 13, 2021.

11. Erwin PC, Brownson RC. The public health practitioner of the future. *Am J Public Health.* 2017;107(8):1227–1232. doi:10.2105/AJPH.2017.303823.

12. MCH Navigator: A Training Portal for MCH Professionals. National Center for Education in Maternal and Child Health. https://www.mchnavigator.org

13. Public Health Innovation Playbook. Public Health National Center for Innovations website. http://www.phnciplaybook.com. Published 2018.

14. Rigolon A, Nemeth J. Green gentrification or "just green enough": Do park location, size and functions affect whether a place gentrifies or not? *Urban Stud.* 2020;57(2):402–420. doi:10.1177/0042098019849380.

15. Government Alliance on Race and Equity. Racial Equity Toolkit: An Opportunity to Operationalize Equity. https://www.racialequityalliance.org/wp-content/uploads/2015/10/GARE-Racial_Equity_Toolkit.pdf. Published September 2015.

15

Using Systems Thinking to Build Preparedness and Response Readiness

Gina Massuda Barnett, Millka Baetcke,
Grace Castillo, and Christina R. Welter

CHAPTER OBJECTIVES

After reading this chapter, the practitioner will be able to:

- Discuss the need to approach emergency preparedness from a systems thinking perspective.
- Articulate the challenges of public health emergency preparedness and response.
- Describe Cook County Department of Public Health's (CCDPH) journey using systems thinking concepts.
- Identify strategies for building an enduring systems thinking approach to preparedness and response.

INTRODUCTION

Coronavirus disease 2019 (COVID-19) has highlighted the opportunity for using systems thinking as a leadership tool in preparing for and responding to an emergency. Addressing both technical and adaptive challenges as well as the need for community-wide and cross-sector responses, systems thinking has been invaluable in helping to diagnose problems, leverage resources, create pathways for communication and coordination, and expose innovative opportunities. Even before COVID-19 and for the past 20 years, Illinois' Cook County Department of Public Health (CCDPH) has approached its public health emergency preparedness and response strategy through the lens of systems thinking. Past systems thinking experiences shaped CCDPH's vision for its COVID-19 response to create an equity-focused, racial justice–centered approach to contact tracing and vaccine distribution.

This chapter is a case study of systems thinking concepts that have guided CCDPH and offers a practical example for others to consider.

THE NEED FOR SYSTEMS THINKING IN PUBLIC HEALTH EMERGENCY AND RESPONSE

While COVID-19 is arguably the largest emergency response event in recent history, there are numerous other examples of emergency preparedness and response over the last century, including H1N1, Ebola, Zika, SARS/MERS, West Nile virus, bioterrorism, HIV/AIDS, and polio. Public health's response performance has hinged in part on its ability to balance and create positive results despite tensions in the public health system or elsewhere. The pandemic has highlighted these tensions, underscoring the need for systems thinking leadership to address public health's preparedness and response challenges.

There are many definitions of systems thinking and ways in which it applies to public health practice and in the context of an emergency. For purposes of the CCDPH case study, we focus on three concepts. First, an important component of systems thinking is understanding diverse community perspectives and situating a problem in the context of its setting.[1] This lets us consider new ways to frame the problem and its solutions that reflect and leverage community assets and challenges to help us practice effective collaboration.[2] Preparing and responding to emergencies requires effective use of public health science in the context of community strengths and resources where content and context expertise must be at least balanced. This is the art and science that best describes the actual practice of public health. COVID-19 underscored this need—where science took a back seat to politics and community concerns. A systems leadership perspective can help meet such a challenge.[3]

Another important systems thinking concept is recognizing both the technical and the adaptive challenges when preparing for and responding to an emergency. A technical challenge is a situation in which the problem and solution can be most easily defined and addressed by existing knowledge, by new knowledge that can be gathered, or by an expert. An adaptive challenge, on the other hand, is complex. There is no clear understanding of the scope, timeframe, and complexity of the problem; the challenge does not have a clear definition and solution; and more than one expert must weigh in. Understanding the distinction between technical and adaptive challenges and framing a given problem and opportunity as an adaptive one require systems thinking. Instead of focusing on what needs to be addressed in the moment, systems thinking helps us understand and make decisions that will have long-lasting, sustainable impact rooted in community and systems strengths.

COVID-19 raised both technical and adaptive challenges. The virus presented us with technical challenges—ones that could be addressed with masks, vaccine provision and acceptance, contact tracing, and community mitigation measures. It also brought the adaptive challenges of recognizing that the disproportionate effects of the pandemic on Black, Latinx, and Indigenous people are rooted in existing health inequities, as well as the need to build community resilience, especially in those populations most affected.

The third systems thinking concept important to preparedness and response is understanding the interrelationships and leverage points that reveal opportunities for maximizing resources and benefits.[1] Response to COVID-19 has been hindered by a resource-poor and fragmented public health infrastructure. The proportion of total health spending has been decreasing since 2000 and falling in inflation-adjusted terms since the Great Recession. Previous to COVID-19, funding for emergency preparedness programs in the last decade was cut in half. In addition, the size of the public health workforce has been reduced significantly: Over the last 10 years, local public health departments lost an estimated 56,360 staff positions due to lack of funding. In 2017, 51% of large local public health departments reported job losses.[4] Taking a systems thinking approach to COVID-19 response presented two important opportunities: First, the response emphasized the importance of using partner assets, expertise, and connections to expand public health's reach and effort. Second, the response provided a strategic window into the need for sustained funding going forward.

Systems thinking in public health emergency preparedness and response is more vital today than ever before. The pandemic has taught us that readiness is not a one-time act but rather an ongoing process. It requires the ability to embrace the complexities and richness of our communities, turning their challenges and strengths into strategies and approaches, "organizing complexity into a coherent story that illuminates the causes of problems and how they can be remedied in enduring ways."[(p128)] Here is the story of how CCDPH employed systems thinking to create and facilitate a community-centered preparedness and response system.

SUBURBAN COOK COUNTY: A WEB OF OPPORTUNITY FOR SYSTEMS CHANGE

The CCDPH is the state-certified health department for nearly all suburban Cook County (SCC), Illinois (excluding Evanston, Oak Park, Skokie, and Stickney Townships, all of which have their own respective state-certified public health departments). SCC is a geopolitically complex region, with 2.5 million people in over 130 municipalities and 30 townships that serve some of the poorest and some of the wealthiest communities in the country. The region's population is increasingly diverse, with the total population of Asian Americans and Pacific Islanders, Blacks, and Hispanics increasing by over 12% between 2010 and 2017 (Chicago Metropolitan Agency for Planning analysis, American Community Survey data, unpublished data, November 2019). While there have been decreases in poverty from 2010 to 2019 across race and ethnicity groups, Black (16.9%) and Hispanic (14.5%) poverty rates in SCC are still twice that of Whites (6.5%; CCDPH analysis of data from U.S. Census Bureau—2000 Census, 2010 Census. U.S. Census Bureau, 2010, 2015–2019 American Community Survey 5-Year Estimates, unpublished data, May 2021). In addition, SCC has a highly disparate, unequal, and fragmented health and social service network and is home to a large number of stakeholders (among them, 20 hospitals, 40 federally qualified health centers, and 143 public school districts with 700 schools; Cook County Department of Public Health [2016], WePlan2020 Suburban Cook County Community Health Assessment and Community Health Improvement Plan, unpublished document, 2016).

The Challenge: Addressing Preparedness Now While Building the Future

In the wake of the September 11, 2001, terrorist attacks and subsequent bioterrorism, CCDPH and other governmental public health agencies received an influx of funding to boost infrastructure for preparing for and responding to acts of bioterrorism. Public health departments were asked, for example, specifically to prepare to receive an emergency shipment of antibiotics for distribution to the public within 48 hours of an identified bioterrorism attack such as anthrax.[5]

While the funding was welcomed, it came with challenges. First, by 2001, CCDPH, like many U.S. public health departments, had experienced significant staffing and resource reductions. While the bioterrorism funds were in part meant to address this, public health officials like chapter authors Christina Welter, Gina Massuda Barnett, and Millka Baetcke recognized that it was impossible to achieve the antibiotic distribution mandate with existing public health resources. The agency did not have sufficient staff and would need support from antibiotic dispensing clinics to cover its jurisdiction. How could CCDPH organize the region's assets and partners for effective public health planning, preparedness, and response?

Second, awareness of and trust in public health in 2001 were limited. As noted in the Institute of Medicine's 1988 report *The Future of Public Health,* the public health system was in disarray.[6] The role of public health was shifting away from providing service and toward an emphasis on addressing more complex population health issues (e.g., chronic disease) through partnerships. In *Betrayal of Trust,* author Laurie Garrett wrote that public health agencies were known for withholding data and information from partners until it was too late.[7] How could CCDPH build trust and value for public health using bioterrorism funding as the vehicle?

Third, there remained growing inequities in health outcomes within CCDPH's jurisdiction. Preparing for bioterrorism was one of many needs of the populations of SCC communities. How could CCDPH leverage bioterrorism funding to build capacity for other disease prevention and control efforts and to address issues of equity?

Systems Thinking Approaches to Understanding the Situation, Exposing Opportunity, Building Trust, and Creating Long-Lasting Systems of All-Hazards Preparedness and Response Systems

Chapter authors Welter, Massuda Barnett, and Baetcke led the CCDPH Community Preparedness and Coordination Unit (CPCU)—now known as the Emergency Preparedness and Response Unit—during its formative years beginning in 2002. Using systems thinking, they reframed bioterrorism as the opportunity to build value for public health in new ways and identified resources and partners to leverage and build community trust through engagement and leadership. Their work in building an all-hazards, cross-sectoral preparedness and response system paved the way for SCC's COVID-19 response. Following are some of the ways in which these leaders applied systems thinking to develop strategic and sustainable approaches to preparedness and response.

Reframe the Technical Problem as an Adaptive Challenge

CPCU broadened the definition of the bioterrorism problem and reframed the challenge from a technical one to an adaptive one, with an eye toward building infrastructure and systems for CCDPH and its jurisdiction. The grant and response deliverables to respond to an act of bioterrorism were unattainable for CCDPH. Reflecting on the disarray in public health and the distrust of public health in general, CPCU chose to explore alternate ways of defining the challenge and opportunity. The team knew that the bioterrorism funding—like most grant funds—would expire. "Public health had to ground ourselves in systems thinking to plan beyond the current issue of bioterrorism," Baetcke says, "and to engage in a longer-term process and vision: It's about how we deal with both current and emerging challenges in the world."

Assess the Possibilities: An Exploration of Community Assets, Connections, and Leverage Points

In 2002 to 2003, CPCU conducted an environmental scan of SCC's strengths, challenges, opportunities, and threats to preparedness and response readiness. The team met with hundreds of partners, including school administrators and nurses, fire and police chiefs, hospital emergency responders, emergency managers, and other key stakeholders at the municipal, county, and state levels. Through informal interviews, they learned about perceptions of public health, its role in preparedness, and the capacities and assets already present. "Principles of qualitative inquiry were applied to get an in-depth understanding of systems in place," says Welter, "and we immediately found that there were many systems in place and opportunities to strengthen public health planning, preparedness, and response." The team also explored jurisdictional methods within the state and across the country.

The survey revealed that SCC had a novel regionalized infrastructure, with overlapping systems and layers of emergency response systems. The more than 130 municipalities within SCC were organized into four regions supported by intergovernmental agencies, referred to as Councils of Government, which provided technical assistance and joint services to their municipal members. Similarly, the Regional Office of Education was the liaison between the hundreds of SCC school districts and the Illinois State Board of Education. Emergency and trauma hospitals were organized into several emergency management services regions. Fire agencies had developed a one-of-a-kind, nationally recognized statewide Mutual Aid Box Alarm System (MABAS)—a regionally organized systems-based resource allocation and distribution network that provided rapid response when a jurisdiction or region was stricken by an overwhelming emergency event. Law enforcement had just begun to develop the Illinois Law Enforcement Alarm Systems (ILEAS),[8] an organizing approach similar to the MABAS[9] network.

The environmental scan also identified gaps and opportunities for CCDPH's role. As noted, SCC is fraught with inequities, and emergency planning and response readiness are no different. Some communities had robust fire and police presence, emergency management support and staffing, school nurses, and other community resources; other communities did not. In addition, the survey revealed that most response systems did not talk with one another. These findings—both the assets and the gaps—stressed the importance of leveraging and building on the tremendous capacity of SCC and the need (or opportunity) to strengthen planning, preparedness, and response coordination across the region.

A New Role: Facilitate Partnerships Through Coordinated Systems and Build Trust and Shared Value

> *"Because outcomes of public health efforts are not immediately tangible, it is often challenging to communicate the value of public health. We have to step back, acknowledge our important role, and highlight our public value effectively." —Gina Massuda Barnett, MPH*

In the event of a large-scale public health emergency, CCDPH is the lead agency in protecting the public's health from communicable disease or undue harm from bioterrorism agents. Acknowledging SCC's inequities and fragmented partnerships, CPCU took a regionalized approach and built a team in which regional emergency response coordinators engaged with multiple response partners while also connecting across SCC. The team worked to develop systems and structures that could be applied to any type of emergency. The outcome was local, regional, and county response systems. "We engaged deeply with these interconnected systems, and this more holistic understanding allowed us to pursue a flexible, coordinated approach," Welter says. "This cohesion and adaptability enabled an all-hazards readiness to share information, conduct joint trainings, run preparedness exercises collaboratively, and build trust across all communities and response structures."

Leading a Multi-Sectoral, All-Hazards Systems Approach in Suburban Cook County: Examples of Success

Localized, Community-Based Planning Teams

One of the first steps in developing a multi-sectoral, all-hazards systems approach in SCC was to start locally and cultivate relationships with the first-responder community and key stakeholders within each SCC region. To do this, CPCU tapped into its training and expertise in community engagement, which involves dynamic relationships, dialogue, and resource sharing, to determine how to organize planning and response teams. This work resulted in the creation of 50 planning teams across SCC, which varied in size and accounted for the established systems and networks (e.g., MABAS divisions) and municipal capacity and resources. Each team included representatives from CCDPH; Cook County Emergency Management Agency; and local emergency management—fire, law enforcement, public works, schools, hospitals, community-based organizations (CBOs), social service agencies, and/or faith-based institutions. With support from their regional emergency response coordinator, the planning teams met regularly to develop their respective local point of dispensing (POD) plan for distribution of pharmaceuticals in response to a bioterrorism event. The vision was to create division planning groups encompassing representatives from local planning teams for three to seven PODs assigned to one of three Regional Planning Oversight Committees representing the north, west, and south SCC regions. While these structures supported local planning, the goal was for each to play a role in systems development and coordination across SCC. While this did occur in some cases, it did not in others. The overall vision, however, turned out to be valuable years later for the COVID-19 response.

First Responder Task Force and Crisis Action Team

In recognition of the need to coordinate across the SCC region, the SCC and CCDPH First Responder Task Force (FRTF) in 2003 began to assist CCDPH in developing operational response plans to biological threats. First responders are critical in addressing large-scale public health events and particularly in assisting CCDPH in preventing and controlling spread of disease. The FRTF was formed for two reasons: (a) to work in partnership with CCDPH to develop and improve response plans and their respective policies, protocols, and procedures that involved first responders, and (b) to serve as a coordinating body through which first responders in SCC would obtain consistent information.

Comprising a leadership team, a general body, and committees, the FRTF was connected to the 50 local planning teams described earlier. It was facilitated by CCDPH and had representation from MABAS, ILEAS, other law enforcement bodies (e.g., the FBI), resource hospitals, dispatch centers, private ambulances, the Councils of Government, Illinois Department of Public Health and Cook County planning team members from the Emergency Management Agency, Sheriff's Policy Department, and Highway Department. The task force addressed crosscutting issues on a strategic level and ensured that vital communications and information were shared. The framework addressed the issue of timely communication of public health data, helped response partners to prepare in advance of an actual emergency, and built trust in shared dialogue.

Following development of the FRTF to support planning and preparedness, CCDPH and the FRTF in 2006 created the First Responder Crisis Action Team (FRCAT) to support response. During the H1N1 outbreak in 2009 to 2010, for example, this team was activated to ensure that all SCC first responders were notified of the potential public health emergency and that unified messages outlining specific response actions were communicated.

An Equity-Based, Regional Approach

As local and regional planning continued in the north, west, and south suburbs, a central challenge was coordination and communication across all 50 PODs in the event of a bioterrorism attack that required all of them to be activated. While this systems change did not come to fruition, efforts made to address the dilemma are good examples of systems thinking.

Activating all PODs simultaneously would create a situation where the north region of SCC, which had higher capacity and more resources, would be unable to assist the other regions, which were expected to require extra resources and support. CCDPH's CPCU worked with the FRTF leadership team and the north SCC region to develop a regional system and had the opportunity to test it in 2009.

The exercise was inspirational. Multiple parties recognized the regional system's potential value and were invested in understanding how to align it with principles of incident command and operationalize it. Through planning and preparing for the exercise, we saw how critical it was for municipalities to act regionally to buffer the effect of various resources being available only in some locales. Focusing on just one or only a few PODs would not build the capacity needed to support less-resourced communities in a large-scale public health emergency; municipal, regionalized cooperation could build the infrastructure and system for responding effectively to any type of emergency, public health or otherwise. Looking beyond the issue of bioterrorism for the first time, CCDPH's CPCU realized that a regionalized, network-based approach connected with local-level change could be applied to other complex public health issues, such as chronic disease.

MOVING FORWARD: APPLYING SYSTEMS CHANGE TO COVID-19 USING LESSONS OF THE PAST

While CCDPH's capacity and the SCC landscape have changed over the last decade, this prior work in preparedness influenced the agency's COVID-19 response. Chapter authors Christina Welter, Gina Massuda Barnett, and Millka Baetcke, who led the CPCU in its early days, returned to support CCDPH in responding to the crisis. Massuda Barnett, deputy director of public health programs for CCDPH and the agency's planning section chief for COVID-19, and Baetcke, a senior consultant on emergency management for Integrated Solutions, were significantly involved. Welter, now faculty at the University of Illinois Chicago School of Public Health and director of its doctoral program in public health leadership, served in technical assistance and lead evaluator roles for the strategic and operational aspects of CCDPH's contact tracing initiative. Fundamentals of CCDPH's actions were: leveraging existing partnerships, networks, and systems and cultivating new ones; honoring authentic community engagement principles at all levels in the system; applying equity as a crosscutting value; and being responsive and adaptive as the situation evolved.

Both contact tracing and vaccine administration were adaptive challenges, and there were several ways in which that work could be undertaken. Positioning equity front and center, CCDPH recognized that earning community trust—especially with people of color—was essential to an effective response that would not exacerbate disparities. The following is a discussion of CCDPH's approach to contact tracing and COVID-19 vaccine administration, the value of systems thinking, and the application of equity principles.

Contact Tracing Initiative as a Community Capacity-Building and Power-Building Endeavor

Lessons learned from its past preparedness and response efforts helped CCDPH to view contact tracing not as a technical task but rather the opportunity to build capacity and systems to address current and future public health issues beyond the pandemic. The agency used contact tracing funds to prevent and control the spread of the virus as well as to cultivate sustainable systems and structures for racial and economic justice. CCDPH worked with partners to advance a collective power-building approach for ongoing collaboration to promote healthy work environments that protect worker rights, health, and safety and help SCC communities thrive. Toward this end, CCDPH invested over $5 million in a 6-month period for two programs within its contact tracing initiative, the Suburban Cook County Worker Protection Program and the Suburban Cook County COVID-19 Community Supports Program. Both programs recognized the value of CBOs as credible, trusted entities and the importance of leveraging existing community assets and infrastructure to share timely and evolving COVID-19 information as well as provide resources to the communities and populations most affected by the pandemic. With a focus on equity, most of the funding was awarded to CBOs located in or near communities hardest hit by COVID-19.

CCDPH and its partners developed a theory of change centered on strategic methods that included diversity, equity, and inclusion; community power; mutually beneficial partnerships; capacity-building; and communications. The theory of change posited that directing resources to where they were most needed, coupled with capacity-building supports, would lead to priority communities and populations sharing their lived experiences and receiving timely, critical messaging and resources. CCDPH, the CBOs, and residents/workers developed tri-directional communication through a co-creation and shared decision-making process. The expectation was that the public health system would be strengthened, with increases in community trust and responsiveness to community needs; mitigation compliance by workplaces and within communities; and changes in individual knowledge, behaviors, and health outcomes—all driving toward an institutionalized, equity-centered system of coordination, collaboration, and decision-making that advances health equity.

To cultivate leadership and sustainability, capacity-building was central to the contact tracing initiative. CCDPH and its partners took a three-pronged approach to enhancing the capacity of CBOs. All CBOs participated in an "equity lab"—a series of three online sessions intended to help these groups augment their knowledge, skills, and resources to meet program deliverables, advance other projects in their organizations and communities, and support their respective Regional Learning and Action Network (RLAN). These RLAN networks brought together individuals from cross-sector organizations to build relationships, provide real-time feedback from priority populations, learn from each other, and leverage resources for sustainable action. CCDPH created RLAN networks to serve as a response structure and a framework in which CCDPH could co-design and co-develop a mutually beneficial network that could be sustained beyond the end of the grant period. Groups could also choose to participate in peer learning. CBOs have had great success, especially with messaging: in March 2021, they disseminated 139,731 messages through various media.

CCDPH's engagement with worker centers illustrates how, by plugging into existing networks and strategically cultivating relationships, CCDPH developed generative solutions. Prior to COVID-19, CCDPH had begun to establish relationships with worker centers—organizations that advocate for workers' rights and changes to workplace conditions that promote health and safety—through the Healthy Work Collaborative convened by the University of Illinois Chicago's Healthy Communities through Healthy Work (HCHW), part of the CDC/NIOSH-funded Center of Excellence for *Total Worker Health*® Center for Healthy Work. While the relationship between CCDPH and two worker centers initially focused on Cook County's minimum wage and earned sick leave ordinances, their enduring strength helped CCDPH with COVID response. When the pandemic hit, the worker centers helped identify workplaces that were being impacted by the virus. They also helped CCDPH develop a clear process for responding to work-based violations by connecting the agency with the office of the Illinois attorney general. Capitalizing on these existing, strong relationships with organizations, and those organizations' relationships with lower-wage, vulnerable workers, is a form of advanced systems change with wide benefit. The shift in CCDPH's collaboration with worker centers had been under way for years and made it easier for the agency to educate workers about workplace violations amid the pandemic. Together with its community partners, CCDPH aims to build mutual capacity and perspective around worker rights both in relation to COVID-19 and more generally. This activity has brought application, compliance, and enforcement together, and would not have been possible without a long-standing commitment to these relationships.

Vaccine Work

As public health's response to COVID-19 shifted to vaccine operations, CCDPH leveraged the systems and relationships developed to support the contact tracing initiative to prioritize and coordinate equity-based mobile vaccination sites. Even with the adaptive challenge of equitably vaccinating the SCC population—while operating within the confines of limited vaccine, limited staffing, and underdeveloped infrastructures—the goal was to vaccinate 70% of SCC's population or 1,750,000 people.

One of the remarkably successful examples of relationships and systems in place supporting public health's COVID-19 vaccination response was the collaboration between CCDPH and private vaccine providers throughout SCC. CCDPH cultivated and leveraged relationships with many private vaccine providers, including federally qualified health centers, nonprofit organizations, and commercial pharmacies, to offer multiple points of vaccine access throughout the region. This allowed for an adaptable and scalable vaccination network that supplemented other vaccination access points in the community. These partnerships expanded CCDPH's capacity to provide vaccinations and to allocate resources in the communities with greatest need.

The same systems that encouraged coordination with CBOs to support COVID-19 education and awareness efforts helped CCDPH address vaccine hesitancy, which was one of the top concerns among CBOs. Feedback from these groups reported residents' desires to learn about vaccination from a medical professional who was a person of color and understood the history of medicine, as well as residents' lack of trust in government and public health. This was an opportunity for CCDPH to be responsive to those voiced needs and opened the door to reimaging power-building and authentic community engagement.

CCDPH also worked closely with the emergency medical systems (EMS) within SCC, as well as with regional MABAS, to identify community resources that could be leveraged to support vaccination efforts. It is important to note that the impetus for the MABAS- and EMS-supported vaccination strategy came from the community partners and not CCDPH. Some better-resourced communities had the capacity to operate local vaccination sites; other communities were able to offer spaces where county and National Guard staff could administer vaccines, providing more access for these populations.

In taking on the adaptive challenge of providing equitable vaccination throughout SCC, CCDPH listened to the communities and provided solutions to align with their unique needs. CCDPH collaborated with large employers and the region's worker centers to provide on-site vaccination and leveraged private-provider linkages to identify and vaccinate homebound residents. With increased vaccine availability and access, CCDPH adapted its goals and response to meet the needs of its constituency. CCDPH strove to ensure equity by working with CBOs to select community venues and events to bring the vaccine to where it was the most familiar, comfortable, and accessible for residents.

CHAPTER SUMMARY

Reflecting on the early days of SCC preparedness and CCDPH's response to COVID-19, there are several lessons learned. First, systems change takes time. Systems thinking is about dealing with challenges in the long term, not just what we are seeing right now. Because of continual change in the landscape that impacts systems change, public health must remain flexible and dynamic. Second, leadership and champions are key to developing and sustaining a systems approach, which can result in systems change. Effective leadership diagnoses a problem more broadly, sets the vision and framework, and empowers all key stakeholders in driving toward the future state. Formal leaders and champions each play important roles in maintaining and cultivating systems change, allowing it to grow and propagate over time. Third, strengthening the public health system and advancing equity require authentic, meaningful engagement with CBOs, sharing power, and ensuring that community and worker voices are elevated and heard. Being authentic, sharing power, and building systems also means going outside of preconceived notions and comfort zones—and it means understanding that the systems built are better than the sum of their parts. Fourth, integrating a method for building capacity—within the local health department and with partners—can have long-lasting impacts. Building a shared vision and a way of operating, coupled with knowledge, skills, and abilities, supports a culture shift. What began in the CPCU set the stage for other CCDPH departments to apply systems thinking to other complex public health challenges.

Key Messages

- Public health is no stranger to emergency preparedness and response. Public health's response performance has hinged in part on its ability to balance and create positive results despite tensions in the public health system or elsewhere. COVID-19 highlighted these tensions, underscoring the need for systems thinking leadership to address public health's preparedness and response challenges.
- Systems thinking in emergency preparedness and response requires: understanding diverse community perspectives and situating a problem in the context of its setting; defining both the technical and the adaptive challenges; and looking for the interrelationship and leverage points in the systems that might expose the opportunities to maximize resources and benefits.
- The CCDPH experience provides a useful case study about applying systems thinking in public health and using lessons from the past to influence the future in meaningful and equity-focused ways.

Tips

- Practice systems thinking before, during, and after an emergency. Even a brief pause to identify the technical and adaptive challenges, explore opportunities, and connect with partners and resources can enhance the response.
- Gather a diversity of perspectives from all levels in the systems and look for the connections. Communities often have networks already in place that are the best pathways for resources and information flow.
- Build partnerships for the long term. These trusting relationships can help maximize resources, expand outreach, and amplify the response in meaningful ways. Often, partners can develop best practices that speak to the community in ways that public health cannot.

Supplemental Resources

- Cook County Department of Public Health: https://cookcountypublichealth.org
- Environmental Scanning: www.upcounsel.com/environmental-scanning
- Theory of Change: www.theoryofchange.org/what-is-theory-of-change
- History of Public Health and Preparedness and Response: Foreman, CH. *Plagues, Products, and Politics: Emergent Public Health Hazards and National Policymaking.* Brookings Institution Press; 1994.

REFERENCES

1. Senge P, Hamilton H, Kania J. The dawn of system leadership. *Stanf Soc Innov Rev.* 2015;13(1):27–33. doi:10.48558/YTE7-XT62.
2. Hayashi C, Soo A. Adaptive leadership in times of crisis. *Prism: J Center Comp Oper.* 2021;4(1):78–86.
3. Baker EL, Irwin R, Matthews G. Thoughts on adaptive leadership in a challenging time. *J Public Health Manag Pract.* 2020;26(4):378–379. doi:10.1097/PHH.0000000000001179.
4. Heifetz RA, Linsky M. A survival guide for leaders. *Harv Bus Rev.* 2002;80(6):65–74, 152. PMID: 12048995.
5. Watson CR, Watson M, Sell TK. Public health preparedness funding: key programs and trends from 2001 to 2017. *Am J Public Health.* 2017;107(S2):S165–S167. doi:10.2105/AJPH.2017.303963.
6. Institute of Medicine. *The Future of Public Health.* The National Academies Press; 1988. doi:10.17226/1091.
7. Garett L. *Betrayal of Trust: The Collapse of Global Public Health.* Oxford University Press; 2003.
8. Illinois Law Enforcement Alarm System (ILEAS). https://www.ileas.org. Accessed June 1, 2021.
9. Mutual Aid Box Alarm System (MABAS). http://www.mabas-il.org/Pages/default.aspx. Accessed June 1, 2021.

Afterword

Golda Philip

Public trust in government—the key social institution for ensuring the health and well-being of individuals—is far from secure.[1] If you have read this book, you likely identify as someone who seeks to catalyze systems change across institutions. If this is you, a lack of public trust and confidence should be of great concern. Without establishing trust, institutions fail to establish legitimacy. Without legitimacy, the effectiveness of institutions and the systems in which they operate is significantly compromised.

Nowhere is trust more important than in public health. Establishing and maintaining the public's trust in health information and corresponding guidance should be a bedrock of public health efforts. The importance of public trust has been evident throughout the phases of the coronavirus disease 2019 (COVID-19) pandemic. Public health systems across the globe rely on members of the public to trust the information and follow the guidance they disseminate in order to contain, mitigate, and recover from the pandemic. At the time this book was in production during the summer of 2021, the Delta variant of COVID-19 was sweeping the globe. Delta infections led to a global surge in cases and a corresponding wave of hospitalizations and deaths, particularly among the unvaccinated. Delta's impact has underscored the global scientific consensus that mass vaccination of populations is key to defeating this pandemic. We also know that public health efforts to vaccinate are dependent on the public's trust—trust in both the vaccine itself and the institutions that produced and promote their use.[2] Thus, public health systems' successes and failures in fighting this pandemic will provide direct insight into our successes and failures in establishing public trust.

The need to establish trust, within and across communities, is more urgent than ever—and more challenging. Recent U.S. survey findings reveal an American public that lacks a high level of trust in key public health institutions. In fact, Americans tend to have higher trust in doctors and nurses than public health institutions, including local, state, and federal government agencies.[3] Reasons for public distrust are many. Widespread misinformation and disinformation—facilitated by advancements in technology and media—have significantly contributed to the challenges governments and associated institutions face as they struggle to be seen as primary arbiters of truth and fact. For communities of color in the United States—particularly Black and Indigenous communities—historical, institutional, and interpersonal discrimination, which was often government-sanctioned, have justifiably resulted in a deep distrust of public health systems and supporting institutions. This distrust is a direct result of decades of segregated medical and public health facilities, forced sterilizations, and violent and involuntary medical treatment and experimentation. Importantly, this distrust is not simply a problem of the past but is one of the present, as medical racism and unequal access to health services persist today.[4]

While the path forward will not be easy, a majority of Americans across all demographic and political groups believe that building trust is still possible.[1] As we think about how to transform public health practice through approaches like systems change, we must acknowledge that building trust in our public health systems will be key to our ability to achieve sustained public health transformation. Relatedly, the only way we are going to establish and maintain this trust is through transformed public health approaches. Transformation is a tall order, and facing the work of institutional and systems transformation is certainly daunting. This book offers public health practitioners a variety of important systems change tools that will help you on your journey. While you can begin your systems change efforts at multiple levels, you may be asking yourself: How will I know where to begin?

From years of work within public health institutions, I offer the following as starting points: recognize and communicate the need for a fundamental shift; allow for pause, reflection, and a clearing of space; and put into place different processes to get different results.

Recognize and communicate the need for a fundamental shift. If you are reading a book on systems change, you may already recognize the fact that most past and current strategies to address some of our most pressing public health challenges, such as the continued existence of health disparities across health conditions, are not working. While *you* may have that understanding, have the leaders in your institution openly acknowledged that reality? Has it been assumed but not publicly stated? It takes both humility and courage for leaders in an organization to acknowledge that what has been done has not been successful and thus requires a fundamental shift in approach. Fundamental shifts are not marginal tweaks to the same program, or using the current "hot topic" words of the day to simply rebrand old efforts. Systems change requires a fundamental shift in approach and an initial step to making that shift is to openly acknowledge the need for it at every level of the organization.

Allow for pause, reflection, and clearing of space. Once you recognize the need for a fundamental shift, you will need to determine a path forward. The day-to-day work of institutions is often deadline-driven, filled with meetings that seem to run into each other and through strings of days, weeks, and years. Programs need to operate, decisions need to be made, deliverables created, services delivered. In many organizations, team retreats are often well-intentioned attempts at team-building but they allow for little meaningful retreat from activity and time for reflection. How often do you and your teams take time to pause long enough to ask, reflect, and answer the question of how or even if your work is making a meaningful impact on the public's health? The more complex the problems you are trying to solve, the longer pause you may need. There are many ways to implement this pause, both formal and informal, but it is only after this kind of reflection that we can begin to truthfully identify the results of our efforts. Every organization I have been part of has engaged in some activities, often long-running activities, that have little to no meaningful result. If this is true for your organization, one next step is to stop doing what's not working. While there may be certain things that must be done regardless of actual impact, perhaps because of law or mandate, these are usually few. Stopping what's not working clears space for you and your teams to invest effort into what does.

Put into place different processes in order to get different results. Once you have cleared space, you can then begin to replace old efforts with innovations. This cannot be an immediate task; it will require process, evaluation, and continuous refining. A key principle in how to change your processes is to change who participates in them. For example, organizations often engage in time and resource-intensive strategic planning processes. Many of these organizations gather stakeholder feedback at the beginning of their strategic planning process and then do the actual planning with internal staff. Is there a way to include stakeholders, both partner organizations as well as individual recipients of your organization's services, throughout the process so that the process itself is transformed and can lead to a new vision for what's needed and possible? Chapters in this book provide practical suggestions for how practitioners can reimagine their efforts through processes that center racial justice; power-sharing (Chapter 2); and meaningful partnerships with communities, coalitions, and non-traditional organizations across different sectors (Chapters 7 and 8). These pages contain critical strategies that will allow for new processes and different, more diverse, stakeholders who will help better define the problems and shift to crafting more sustainable solutions. Taken together, these strategies will allow for a reconceptualization of public health capacity from the workforce within individual public health organizations to a far stronger and sustainable workforce that harnesses the energy and input of impacted communities as well as the organizational strength of cross-sectoral institutions. It is this magnitude of force that is required for systems change.

One important note: The same principle of changing processes to get different results also applies to the work of internal individual and team development. The book's chapters on interpersonal leadership (Chapter 5) and team development (Chapters 6 and 7) provide you with important frameworks and action steps to reimagine processes within your organizations and teams. Indeed, transformation of public health practice work needs to be done with integrity—transforming public health practice on the outside through organizations that have committed to the process of transformation on the inside.

The work of systems change is the work of transformation, and it cannot be completed in a single planning cycle or fiscal year. This work requires a structured commitment to the ongoing process of seeing, listening, acting, and reflecting for yourselves, your teams, and your organizations. And for true systems change to happen, you need to commit to all levels of this process in authentic community with those closest to the conditions you are trying to improve or the issues you are trying to solve. Through this process, you will (re)form personal and institutional relationships upon which systems are built, establish trust, and cocreate solutions to build a healthier world.

DISCLAIMER

This article was written by the author in her personal capacity. The opinions expressed in this article are the author's own and do not reflect the view of the Health Resources Services Administration, the Department of Health and Human Services, or the U.S. government.

REFERENCES

1. Rainie L, Keeter S, Perrin A. Trust and Distrust in America. Pew Research Center; July 22, 2019. https://www.pewresearch.org/politics/2019/07/22/trust-and-distrust-in-america/.
2. Organisation for Economic Co-Operation and Development. Enhancing Public Trust in COVID-19 Vaccination: The Role of Government. https://www.oecd.org/coronavirus/policy-responses/enhancing-public-trust-in-covid-19-vaccination-the-role-of-governments-eae0ec5a/. Published May 10, 2021.
3. Robert Wood Johnson Foundation. The Public's Perspective on the United States Public Health System. https://cdn1.sph.harvard.edu/wp-content/uploads/sites/21/2021/05/RWJF-Harvard-Report_FINAL-0513212.pdf. Published May 2021.
4. Nuriddin A, Mooney G, White AIR. Reckoning with histories of medical racism and violence in the USA. *The Lancet*. 2020, October 3;396:949–951. https://www.thelancet.com/action/showPdf?pii=S0140-6736%2820%2932032-8.

Index

de Beaumont

BOLD SOLUTIONS FOR HEALTHIER COMMUNITIES

Founded in 1998, the de Beaumont Foundation advances policy, builds partnerships, and strengthens public health to create healthier communities where people can achieve their best possible health.

OUR MISSION

We advance policy, build partnerships, and strengthen public health to create communities where people can achieve their best possible health.

The de Beaumont Foundation creates and invests in bold solutions that improve the health of communities across the country. We believe that every person should have the opportunity to achieve their best health, regardless of where they live.

Our vision is a nation where every person in every community has the opportunity to achieve their best possible health.

OUR FOCUS

POLICY:
We advance policies that improve community health, so that current and future generations can benefit from changes enacted by today's leaders.

PARTNERSHIPS:
We build partnerships, often among unlikely allies, so that leaders can achieve the shared goal of creating healthier communities.

PEOPLE:
We create practical solutions that strengthen the public health system and workforce, so that professionals are equipped to make their communities healthier.

OUR PROGRAMS

Our programs and investments strengthen the public health system, facilitate collaboration, and provide practical tools to improve the health of all Americans.

CityHealth | Policy solutions to help local leaders improve the health of their communities.
Website: https://www.cityhealth.org/

PH WINS | The only nationally representative survey of government public health professionals.
Website: https://debeaumont.org/programs/ph-wins/

40 Under 40 in Public Health | Recognition program for leaders who are improving community health through innovation solutions.
Website: https://debeaumont.org/40-under-40/2019-2/

BEAM | A certificate program in business skills for public health professionals.
Website: https://debeaumont.org/programs/beam/

Big Cities Health Coalition (BCHC) | A powerful coalition of health leaders from 30 of the nation's largest cities.
Website: https://www.bigcitieshealth.org/

Practical Playbook | Tips and lessons to form partnerships between public health and primary care.
Website: https://www.practicalplaybook.org/

The BUILD Health Challenge | Public health, healthcare, and community organizations working to improve health.
Website: https://buildhealthchallenge.org/

PHRASES | Tools for public health professionals to communicate more effectively to form partnerships.
Website: https://debeaumont.org/programs/phrases/

deBeaumont.org

deBeaumontFoundation
@deBeaumontFndtn
de-Beaumont-Foundation
@deBeaumontFndtn

Printed in the United States
by Baker & Taylor Publisher Services